DATE DUE

APR 12 2013	

BRODART, CO.   Cat. No. 23-221-003

Straight Talk
about Psychological Testing
for Kids

Straight
Talk about
Psychological
Testing for
Kids

Ellen Braaten

Gretchen Felopulos

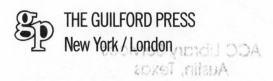

THE GUILFORD PRESS
New York / London

© 2004 The Guilford Press
A Division of Guilford Publications, Inc.
72 Spring Street, New York, NY 10012
www.guilford.com

The information in this volume is not intended as a
substitute for consultation with healthcare professionals.
Each individual's health concerns should be evaluated by
a qualified professional.

Printed in the United States of America

This book is printed on acid-free paper.

Last digit is print number: 9 8 7 6 5 4 3 2 1

Library of Congress Cataloging-in-Publication Data

Braaten, Ellen B.
    Straight talk about psychological testing for kids / Ellen B.
Braaten, Gretchen Felopulos.
        p. cm.
    Includes bibliographical references and index.
    ISBN 1-57230-787-0 (pbk.) — ISBN 1-57230-948-2 (hard)
    1. Psychological tests for children—Popular works.
    I. Felopulos, Gretchen. II. Title.
    RJ503.5.B73 2004
    618.92′89075—dc21

                                        2003010343

For the most important people in my life—
my husband, Eric, and children, Hannah and
Peter. I couldn't have done it without you.

—EB

For my husband, Paul, and our children, Theo,
Chloë, and our daughter waiting for us in
China. I love you all with all my heart.

—GF

Contents

Acknowledgments

Even though we were fortunate to be able to work together on this project, we found that two heads were often not enough in trying to complete a book. We relied on many people over the course of the two years that it took to finish the work, and we'd like to take this chance to thank them all for their help and support.

As two full-time moms with careers, we couldn't have pulled this off without the help of our wonderful husbands, who put in extra time with the kids while we were writing, talking, rewriting, talking. . . . We really appreciate you!

Our editors at The Guilford Press, Christine Benton and Kitty Moore, have been outstanding, and we thank them for their enthusiasm for this project. Kitty nurtured this project from the start, and Chris has handled our manuscript with care, insight, and great skill.

Along the way, various people have helped move this project from idea to fruition. Bonnie Ohye was gracious enough to put us in touch with the right people at Guilford, and Ross Greene advised us from the start on the business aspects of book writing and gave us the lead on our agent, Wendy Lipkind. The members of Anne Fischel's writing group were empathic listeners who encouraged us when we became discouraged. We're also grateful to Chris McCarthy, Molly Battle, Gretchen Timmel, and Roxie Billings for help with all sorts of important details along the way.

The legal information in Chapter Two was reviewed by Eileen Hagerty, an outstanding and dedicated education lawyer with the esteemed Boston-based law firm Kotin, Crabtree & Strong. She put in a lot of time editing the text, and we are grateful for her comments and revisions.

Thanks to all our colleagues at the Psychology Assessment Center and in Child Psychiatry at Massachusetts General Hospital. You are a talented and inspiring group to work with, and we appreciate all your input and suggestions, most of which we incorporated into the book.

As our two minutes are almost up, we'd finally like to thank our families and friends for their love and encouragement over the years— you made us believe we could do it, and we did!

**Straight Talk
about Psychological Testing
for Kids**

Introduction

"My child has reading problems—how can I find out if she's dyslexic?"

"My teenage son has become withdrawn and irritable—could he be depressed? How will I know?"

"How can we figure out whether our five-year-old is ready to start kindergarten?"

These very different questions have a common answer: a testing evaluation. As two clinical psychologists who do hundreds of testing evaluations a year, we talk with parents of widely different children who share similar concerns. The decision to have your child undergo testing is a difficult one, because parents typically know little about the process and just as little about where to go for answers. The purpose of this book is to fill that gap: to respond to a broad range of questions and to support and guide you through procedures that are often confusing for both you and your child but that need not be so stressful. With 15 to 20 percent of all school-age children referred for testing each year, there are literally millions of parents like you seeking answers. We hope you'll find them here.

The parents we meet on a daily basis are concerned about their children's development. Sometimes they have agonized over whether to pursue testing because they were reluctant to have their children "labeled." Other parents have actively sought diagnoses for their children. Some were referred by their schools or pediatricians and are confused as to why their children needed testing in the first place. Whatever the origin of their questions, all the parents we meet have one concern: their children's welfare. Will their children be able to learn like other children do? If their children prove to have a disability, are treatments available for it? Why are their children struggling in school or with life in general? In this book we hope to show how and when educational, neuropsychological, and psychological testing can answer these questions. These assessments, all of which should be performed by qualified professionals called *psychologists,* are the focus of the book, although we include some information on evaluations in speech and language, occupational therapy, and physical therapy, as well.

If you're currently considering having your child tested, you may find yourself surprised at how ill prepared you feel to enter the testing process or to interpret and use the test results. After all, many children you know of have probably been tested, so you know how common these procedures are. One reason for the mystery surrounding these tests is that it is unethical for psychologists to describe tests in enough detail to jeopardize the validity of the test. Also, tests, and the scores generated from them, can be quite difficult to understand and therefore difficult for professionals to explain. There is also considerable confusion regarding the terms used among schools and private settings, such as clinics or hospitals. For example, school systems tend to refer to "psychological testing" as an assessment of intelligence, whereas outside psychologists usually regard psychological testing as an evaluation of a person's emotional functioning and personality traits. Because of inconsistent terminology, it can be challenging to talk about "testing" in a clear, uniform manner. We have attempted to do that, though, and we point out the areas of debate and confusion as we go along so that you are aware of these.

How Should You Use This Book?

Parents today play an increasingly important role in their children's educational development. As a parent, therefore, you are your child's first and best advocate. Your influence ranges from helping to obtain an accurate diagnosis to locating services and setting positive and appropriate expectations for your children to clarifying issues of school placement and arranging for appropriate extracurricular activities. You are no longer viewed as passive recipients of professional advice. Instead, you are likely to be considered equal partners in the development of treatment and educational programs for your children. But you need to be informed if you are to do a good job.

Our approach to informing you is to take you through the testing process from start to finish. We start with concerns you might have when you first think your child may need testing and proceed through the evaluation, possible diagnosis, and treatment decisions. The information in this book comes from a wealth of scientific research and is supported by our own clinical experience. We have placed particular emphasis on your legal rights to have your child evaluated through the public school system—something that every child is entitled to by law but that many parents don't even know about.

To get the most complete picture, we suggest you start at the beginning and more or less read through to the end of the book, but the point you have reached in the testing process when you open up this book may determine the optimal reading sequence for you. Perhaps your child has already been evaluated, but you need information on how to understand the testing report. In that case, your most urgent need might be for the information in Chapter Five. Or your child may be about to begin an evaluation for a certain disorder, say dyslexia, and you want to be sure the psychologist is going to use the kinds of tests most helpful in assessing this concern. In this case, Chapter Six could be your best starting point. Please just don't make it your ending point, too. The rest of the book contains useful information about your rights and other matters that you may not even be aware of, so at least skim through the other sections as well.

Though we feel this book has many uses, it is *not* intended to train you in the methods of testing nor to enable you to determine exactly which tests the professional you are working with should use. By choosing a respected and well-trained clinician (a process discussed in Chapter Three), you will help ensure that your child receives the best possible evaluation, with appropriate tests and recommendations. We hope that reading this book will also help you understand the tests used in your child's evaluation, what the results mean, and how to make sure your child gets the necessary help that has been recommended based on the test results.

How the Book Is Organized

Part I of this book, "Where Do I Begin?," discusses the preliminaries: How do you know your child needs testing? Where do you begin? How do you find a competent professional? We discuss how to initiate the evaluation and the pros and cons of having your child tested within or outside of the school system. We discuss the cost of testing and issues of insurance coverage. To make the information as relevant to you as possible, we present cases of real children going through the evaluation process, in school and privately. The number of professionals available to test children can be quite overwhelming to a parent. We describe the persons who are qualified to do testing, as well as those who do not perform psychological testing but who are often involved in the process. We also describe how to go about finding a competent person and discuss what to do when you feel the professional was not as skilled as you would have liked, as well as when it is appropriate to seek a second opinion.

Part II, "A Practical Guide to Commonly Used Tests," provides information about the tests themselves. We present brief descriptions of the most common tests so that you can know how the tests used for your child will help the clinician determine the child's strengths and weaknesses and also so that you may participate in decisions about which tests to give (though, again, this book is not intended to train you to dictate which tests must be used). We introduce and explain intelligence, achievement, and neuropsychological tests, as well as tests of emotional functioning. Some of the most frequent sources of confusion for parents come from the overwhelming number of facts and figures included in a typical test report. We explain, in simple terms, the most frequent types of test scores that you will encounter. Because many of these tests compare an examinee's performance with that of a norm group (also known as a *comparison group*), we discuss why this type of measurement is important. We provide simple definitions for terms such as *percentiles*, *standard scores*, and *scaled scores* and discuss whether tests are reliable or susceptible to change. In our experience, test scores are the area that parents are most confused about but least likely to question.

Part III, "Common Childhood Disorders," describes the most common disorders for which a child would undergo testing. We've learned that parents want specific information about their child's possible diagnosis but also have questions about why their child was not given a particular diagnosis. We typically hear questions such as "How do you know it's ADHD and not dyslexia?" or "There are so many symptoms that are the same for autism and Asperger syndrome, so how do I know you gave my child the right diagnosis?" This section discusses the symptoms of the most common disorders, using case examples to describe the tests typically used to evaluate each disorder. Each chapter provides an answer to the question "How do I know the psychologist gave my child the right tests?" It also provides information on appropriate treatment strategies for each disorder, as well as resources for you and your child. Throughout the book we provide reassurance, encouragement, and general support for parents going through this often confusing and stressful experience, and we also give more specific resources, such as books, Web sites, support networks, and advocacy groups, at the end of each chapter in this section. Arriving at the decision that your child needs testing is difficult enough. Finding needed support once a diagnosis has been made is essential.

We hope that you find this book supportive, helpful, and useful. Because we want every family we work with to have this knowledge yet find that there isn't always enough time to cover it all, we have written it down for present and future reference. And, for the children and parents we will never meet but are thoughtfully aware of, we hope this book will give you the answers you need to get the help you deserve.

Part 1

Where Do I Begin?

One

How Do I Know My Child Needs Testing?

For the third night in a row, nine-year-old Philip was in tears. Two months into the fourth grade, he was complaining about homework and, even worse, starting to say such things as, "I'm stupid" and "I hate school!" When his parents asked him what was wrong, Philip told them that the work was too hard and that he couldn't understand the assignments. It was true: When his mother tried to help him with his reading work for the week, she saw that he could not read the larger words that had begun to show up in his fourth-grade work. Because of this, he couldn't always understand the material and wasn't able to answer the questions correctly. His parents were confused. Philip seemed very bright. He had learned to read more slowly than his brothers, but he hadn't had any real problems with schoolwork until now. What was going on?

Zach's mother wasn't surprised when she got a call from his first-grade teacher. After all, he had had trouble in preschool with Circle Time, and now Zach was being asked to sit down and learn for most of the school day. Before kindergarten, his pediatrician had said that he would grow out of it and that he was simply immature and rather active. Evidently, Zach's first-grade teacher felt that something more was wrong; she was concerned that he wasn't learning as much as the other students because he wasn't able to pay attention for very long. She also said that Zach had begun to be a distraction in class and was having trouble switching from one activity to another. Zach's parents had already seen the pediatrician about these concerns. Now what were they supposed to do?

Nicole had been looking forward to high school for a long time, but now, in ninth grade, she seemed miserable. The first few months had gone smoothly, and Nicole had become busy with school activities and social events. Now, after the winter break, she was irritable and had stopped going to games and hanging out with friends as she used to do. Furthermore, her grades had started to decline; when her parents asked her about this, she said she didn't care and added, "What's the point of going to school anyway?" The family had a history of depression, and Nicole's mother wondered if she was depressed. Nicole's father chalked it all up to "typical adolescent behavior" and said not to worry. The school guidance counselor wondered whether Nicole might have a learning disability that hadn't been noted before and recommended a testing evaluation. What was the right thing to do? Who could help?

As an only child, Alexandria hadn't had much practice socializing with other kids. At least that's how her parents had always understood her preference for playing by herself. But when she entered preschool, her lack of interest in other children began to worry both her parents and the teachers. Was she just shy, or could there be something wrong? How could they find out?

Perhaps like these parents, you've found that there's something "not quite right" with your child. Although it's true that parents *do* tend to worry about their kids more than they need to, it is also true that parents' intuition is often right about concerns that others, including pediatricians and teachers, do not always pick up on till later, if at all. Our culture tends to underestimate parents' ability to figure out what their child needs, even though, ironically, it's the parent who knows the child best. What we hear frequently is that Mom or Dad knew that their child needed some help *but didn't know how or where to get it.* So this chapter and the rest of this book are intended to give you the information you need to find your child the help he deserves.

The tool or method for figuring out specifically what your child needs and why isn't new, but we find that parents do not generally know about its existence. We're talking about a *testing evaluation*—developmental, psychological, neuropsychological, speech and language, occupational therapy, physical therapy, and other assessments. These terms may not make complete sense to you right now, but the various types of evaluations just mentioned can tell you the nature and severity

Common Types of Testing Evaluations: What They Include

Terminology used for types of evaluation can vary, and the names of specific tests are diverse. What follows are the most common terms, those you're most likely to hear. Details that will explain more fully what the evaluations are intended to produce, how the individual tests are administered, and what you can expect are presented in Chapter Four.

Neuropsychological Evaluation: A test battery designed to measure a child's cognitive skills and brain functioning in areas such as intelligence, attention, memory, learning, and visual perceptual skills. Tests typically given include an intelligence measure, such as the WISC-III; achievement/academic tests, such as the WIAT-II or the Woodcock–Johnson to look for learning disabilities; language tests, such as the Boston Naming Test or the PPVT-III; visual–motor tests, such as the VMI or Rey–Osterrieth Complex Figure Test; tests of memory and executive functions, such as the NEPSY, WRAML, and CMS, and neuromotor tests such as Finger Tapping or Grooved Pegboard.

Educational/Achievement Evaluation: A test battery specifically for measuring a child's academic skills in decoding, reading comprehension, spelling, math, and writing. An intelligence measure should also be given to compare the child's potential (intelligence level) with her achievement scores. Common tests used include the Woodcock–Johnson, the WIAT-II, and WRAT3.

Psychological Evaluation: A test battery for assessing a child's emotional, social, and behavioral functioning and personality traits. Tests often include the Rorschach, TAT, drawings, sentence completion tests, self-report measures such as the Children's Depression Inventory and the MMPI for adolescents, and parent-completed measures such as the Child Behavior Checklist or the BASC.

Developmental Evaluation: A test battery such as the Bayley Scales of Infant Development, administered before age four, that gives information about a young child's level of development in language skills, motor skills, cognitive skills, and social skills.

of and appropriate treatment for your child's particular area of weakness or difficulty. Testing helps to diagnose a certain problem such as a learning disability, to clarify what is wrong (is it ADHD or depression?), and to provide strategies for school and home geared to help the child function better.

Each type of testing evaluation requires a fully trained, specialized professional who takes a full history of your child and the problems the child is having, which you provide in an interview or on intake forms. The evaluator then uses clinical observation, a combination of tests, and consultation with other providers, such as teachers and therapists, to gather a wealth of information about your child and the child's functioning. Next the evaluator compares your child's behavior, test scores, and history with those of same-age peers to figure out if the child is substantially stronger or weaker in any given area. Usually some type of diagnosis, or formal label, is given to account for the concerns that brought you to the evaluation in the first place. Terms such as *autism*, *dyslexia, hypotonia*, and *major depression* are clinical diagnoses that different evaluators may provide, depending on whether or not your child meets the criteria for the particular diagnosis.

When can testing help? We've broken concerns up into various categories, though many of them overlap. See if you have any of the concerns listed in the following section about your child. If so, we take you through the process of getting the right kind of testing evaluation, in the right place, and with the right professional. We also help you understand the reports better by explaining what the tests do, and we

Criteria refer to the various characteristics or symptoms of a given syndrome, disability, or other type of diagnosis.

give you resources and strategies for helping your child once you get the testing evaluation done. We even help you talk with your child about the results—after all, the more she understands about herself, the more accepting she will be of the interventions.

When Testing Can Help

Testing is often used to help provide an explanation for a problem your child has. Testing is not always necessary for understanding what is wrong, but in many cases it proves essential for an accurate diagnosis and an appropriate treatment plan. Difficulty with writing, for example, could be attributable to a number of problems, such as fine-motor muscle weakness, visual–motor integration delays, problems generating ideas, organization difficulties, or inattention. Without the right kind of testing, you won't know what the cause of the problem is nor whether it's possible to eradicate the cause and thereby eliminate the problem or, if not, what kind of intervention will improve your child's success with writing. If the child does not receive a formal diagnosis of a learning disability or emotional disorder, he may not be eligible for services through the school system. It's important to remember that a diagnosis doesn't necessarily guarantee that your child will receive special education services or accommodations, because he may not need them. For example, Todd was diagnosed with bipolar disorder, which was managed effectively with medication and therapy; therefore, no school-based services were warranted.

Even if a child has already been diagnosed with a certain disorder, such as Asperger syndrome, the results of a good testing evaluation will almost always yield more specific information that can enhance the potential for a prescribed treatment to help your child. When a child has a constellation of problems, a testing evaluation can shed light on their relative severity and possible connections among them, helping to reveal any co-occurring disorders (such as the presence of a learning disability in a child who has already been diagnosed with ADHD) or assisting a practitioner in determining which problems should be addressed in treatment. It can also be helpful in highlighting cognitive and emotional strengths that can further augment or guide interventions.

Though we may be biased—because we have seen so many examples of how testing can assist in diagnosis and treatment of children—we believe that testing evaluations are useful in assessing and understanding the majority of the concerns described in the following paragraphs. Check them over and then consult with your pediatrician about any that apply to your child. Although you may not be referred for testing right away, it will be important for your pediatrician to make a note of the observed problem(s) and to figure out what intervention, if any, is needed.

Language and Speech Skills

Speech refers to the production of sounds that make up words and sentences, whereas *language* means the use of words and sentences to communicate needs, ideas, and feelings. Although there can be a lot of variability in exactly when each child begins to babble, say single words, or put together a few words, you are right to be concerned if you have noticed the following:

Infant/Toddler

- Has trouble sucking or swallowing
- "Overstuffs" his or her mouth
- Isn't babbling by around 10 months
- Isn't using single words by age 15–18 months
- Is using only one or two words at a time by age three
- Is not understandable to others outside the family by age three
- Doesn't seem to understand what you are saying by age two and a half
- Seems to "tune out" or fails to listen consistently by age three
- Does not start conversations but only responds to others by age three
- Repeats what is heard from others, from TV, and so forth, rather than responding
- Drools or slurps saliva often at age three
- Has trouble drinking properly from cups, uncapped water bottles, and the like by age three

Preschooler

- Words come out jumbled or in poor order by age four
- Gives only brief responses to open-ended questions by age four
- Replies do not relate to the questions asked by age four
- Can't tell you what a story was about by age four
- Has difficulty answering questions such as "what?" and "when?" and "where?" at four
- Can't articulate (make sounds accurately) clearly by age five
- Still talks a lot about irrelevant topics or strays from the subject often at age five
- Can't answer "how" questions by age five
- Can't follow a two-step direction such as "Go upstairs; get your shoes, please" at age five

School Age and Up

- Seems frustrated by problems finding words or communicating
- Often mishears what is said

- Has trouble getting the gist of jokes or idioms such as "You're pulling my leg!" by age six
- Has a continually scratchy or rough, nasal, or squeaky voice

Though this is a long list, it is not complete. You may have other speech or language concerns about your child that are not included here. We strongly encourage you to talk to your friends, pediatrician, and teachers. We also recommend that you do some of your own research on-line or at the library.

If you and/or someone else in your child's life decides that a speech or language concern deserves professional attention, see a *speech and language pathologist,* a trained professional who will use testing to evaluate your child's speech and language development as compared with that of same-age peers and provide the necessary treatment.

Motor Skills

There are many types of motor skills, but the ones that tend to be talked about the most with respect to children's development are fine-motor skills and gross-motor skills. *Fine-motor skills* refer to the tasks carried out mainly by your fingers and hands—picking up small objects, holding a spoon or fork, grasping a pencil, using scissors, writing and drawing, tying shoelaces. *Gross-motor skills* include large-muscle-related abilities, such as walking, running, jumping, balancing, eye–hand coordination, and riding a bike.

As with most other things, no two kids will probably achieve the same fine- or gross-motor skill at the same time. However, some guidelines can help you determine at about what point on the developmental trajectory your child's motor skills should be. You should talk to your pediatrician if you notice any of the following concerns:

Infant/Toddler

- Does not attempt to reach for objects by three to six months
- Cannot hold his head upright by four months
- Does not grasp objects with her whole hand by six to eight months
- Is not sitting up by ten months
- Cannot use a pincer grip (thumb and forefinger to pick up small objects) by about one year
- Is not walking by eighteen months

- Can't hold a pencil or crayon well enough to scribble by eighteen months
- Can't throw a toy or ball by age two
- Is not running by age two and a half
- Isn't going up stairs by age two and a half
- Has problems with balance at any age over two years
- Can't jump with two feet off the ground at age three
- Has trouble holding his fork or spoon by age two and a half to three
- Is excessively clumsy at any age over three
- Walks or runs awkwardly at any age over three

Preschooler/School Age and Up

- Doesn't alternate feet on the stairs by age four
- Has trouble holding a seated position at a table without slouching or shifting a lot
- Isn't riding a tricycle or bike with training wheels by age five
- Has trouble with the scissors at age five or older
- Has excessive difficulty writing her name or can't write it legibly by age five
- Writes letters or numbers illegibly at age five to six
- Has difficulty with playing sports (e.g., kicking the ball, catching)
- Has weak muscle tone or low stamina at any age

We certainly haven't covered all the possible delays or problems here, so you should really discuss any concerns you have with respect to your child's motor skills with her doctor. There are a few different kinds of professionals who may evaluate and treat your child for potential weaknesses, including *orthopedists*, *occupational therapists*, or *physical therapists*. Your child may also need to see a *neurologist* to determine if there is anything more pervasive or broad affecting your child's development.

Social Skills

Social skills have received less attention than other developmental abilities, but they are essential to your child's functioning and well-being. With some children, social difficulties are obvious, such as the seven-

Q: *I am in a toddler play group with my son, who is now two years old. We have met with the other children and their mothers for about a year now, and I have started to worry that my child isn't doing a lot of the things that the other kids his age can do. He started walking a few months after all the others, and now many of the two-year-olds are putting together a few words to make sentences while my son still babbles. My pediatrician said she is not too concerned but that she would support a testing referral if I wanted to make sure everything was all right. Could testing really tell me much? Would it be stressful for my little boy?*

A: It's hard not to make comparisons between our children and others. Because you are clearly concerned, even though your son's doctor is not, we suggest you follow up on your maternal instincts. Up until your child is three years old, he is eligible to be evaluated by your town's Early Intervention (EI) program (for more information on this, see Chapter Two). Your child may receive a general developmental screen, such as the Bayley Scales of Infant Development or the Denver Developmental Screening Test. Because motor and language skills have been a worry, he may also get more specific tests to look at his gross-motor skills, fine-motor skills, and early language skills. The testing process is often fun for toddlers, as toys are used to help the evaluators learn about their skills. You should also be allowed to be present for the testing, as this will help your son feel more comfortable. Your input will be critical in figuring out if there is a problem; if so, you will be glad you did not wait any longer, because research shows that the earlier you intervene, the better the child does.

---

year-old boy who tries to engage other kids by banging them over the head with his plastic baseball bat or the ten-year-old girl who will play only by herself. But with others, social skill problems may be more subtle, such as the child who can't make eye contact with people when interacting or the kid who can't seem to figure out what's going on when he's in a group.

Parents are usually the first to pick up on social skill delays because they're the ones who see their kids interacting with others during free play. Sometimes it's hard to convince others that something's not quite right in this area, mainly because there are few hard and fast rules about social development. For the most part, though, we expect children to become interested in others during the first few months of life, and this interest should keep growing if all goes well. During the toddler years kids will typically start to play with other toddlers, often doing a similar task side by side rather than together; this is usually referred to as "parallel play." By age four and older, children usually shift to cooperative or shared play, in which they have a common play theme and carry out the activity together. It is typical for kids over four to move between parallel and cooperative play, at times even choosing to play by themselves. As a culture, though, we need to be very careful not to let the advances of technology cause widespread isolation among our children, given their common interest in computers and video games. We have seen a real surge of children who think they are being "social" by talking on-line with friends or playing video games next to a buddy for hours; however, these kids often eventually find that they are less physically active, lonely, and generally unhappy as a result of this loss of real human contact.

The same effect occurs for children who have social skill impairments for one reason or another. They are often less active, feel alienated, and become depressed as a result of their difficulties forming relationships with their peers. We strongly encourage you to trust your instincts when it comes to social problems in your child, because these weaknesses are as important to address as others—sometimes more so. Though the possibilities are vast, we've listed a few of the more common social skill difficulties that we see:

Toddler and Up

- Has problems making and keeping eye contact with you or others
- Seems to be uninterested in playing with others, especially by age three
- Doesn't engage in pretend play by age three to four
- Engages only in "play" that involves repeating a story or video theme
- Has problems figuring out how to join in with other kids
- Tends to miss or misunderstand what is meant by others' behavior (often called "problems reading social cues")
- Engages in aggressive or violent play at three and up
- Has an obsessive interest in one topic but a lack of creative playing (e.g., loves dinosaurs and knows every fact about them but can't enact a play scene with them)

- Frequently avoids or shows outright fear of social situations (birthday parties, play dates, the park, school)
- Has difficulty carrying on the natural rhythm of conversation or play
- Shows a lack of social responsiveness to you or others (e.g., does not respond when her name is called; does not acknowledge a child who comes into the room)
- Has a rigid or bossy style with peers that affects his social acceptance

If you should become concerned about any of these issues or one that we haven't covered, again we encourage you to start by talking with your pediatrician. The doctor may refer you to one of several types of professionals, including *child psychologists, developmental pediatricians,* or *speech and language therapists*. When Alexandria's doctor learned about the parents' and teachers' concerns regarding her social skills, he referred them to a child psychologist, who then completed a full evaluation that included some testing. The evaluation first helped the psychologist to figure out the specific nature or cause of Alexandria's social impairment and then to give strategies or recommendations for ways to help.

Learning

For school-age children, learning is probably the most common type of concern. Sometimes parents or teachers catch a learning problem, or *disability,* early, such as in kindergarten or first grade. But because some kids are able to compensate for a while, often these problems are not diagnosed until much later. Philip, for example, didn't show major signs of a problem until fourth grade. Looking back, his mom could recall that he had learned to read with more difficulty than his siblings had, but otherwise he had been doing pretty well. He was a bright child and was able to use other skills to make up for his weaker ones until the material simply became too tough. That's the reason that, even though he was likely born with the problem that caused his learning disability, it wasn't diagnosed until age nine or so.

Although there are many different types of learning disabilities (we've covered the most common ones in Part III of this book), in general you are wise to pursue a testing evaluation if you notice any of the following:

Preschool and Up

- Has problems with rhyming and trouble learning letters and their sounds by age six
- Has difficulty paying attention or following directions
- Experiences frustration doing grade-level work at any age
- Has gaps in skills or inconsistent grades
- Has memory and organization problems
- Experiences a decline in grades or school performance
- Has consistent problems getting homework done
- Routinely runs out of time on tests
- Tells you he hates school or refuses to go

These are very general concerns, but fundamentally they apply to the different kinds of learning problems a child may have. After talking with your child's pediatrician and teachers, you will probably be referred to a *child psychologist*, a *neuropsychologist*, or the school's special education department for an evaluation.

Q: *Our son turns five in August, but we aren't sure whether he is ready to start kindergarten. He passed the public school's readiness screening, but he seems to have more difficulty than other kids his age staying focused on games and other activities. Would a testing evaluation help us make this decision?*

A: Many parents struggle with the decision about when to have their child start kindergarten, especially if he has a birthday near the entrance age cutoff date (e.g., he must be five by September 1). To some extent these entrance dates are arbitrary, considering that many children have the cognitive skills and social readiness to begin kindergarten by age five whereas others need an extra year to develop these abilities. Although the school's screening test gives you some information about your child's basic skills, you as the parent know your child best and are the most equipped to make the decision about when your child should start school.

Many other factors are important to consider besides your son's knowledge of shapes and colors. For example, can he sit for up to fifteen minutes to do a quiet activity such as listening to a story or coloring? Is he able to get along with other children in cooperative play, or does he prefer to play by himself? Does he tend to get aggressive with peers? How well does he deal with frustration—does he have tantrums, or can he use his words to tell how he is feeling? Does he seem to be emotionally young for his age (does he cling to you or become clearly distressed when you leave)? Is he more dependent on you than other kids his age seem to be on their parents? Does he have trouble recognizing or remembering things that you would expect him to know by now?

Although many children who have been successful in kindergarten have had one or two of the preceding concerns, you may want to give some serious thought to keeping your son in preschool for one more year if he has a few cognitive, social, and/or emotional "red flags" that indicate a lack of readiness right now. Remember, although kindergarten does not require kids to do a lot of sitting and thinking, first grade is right around the corner. Talk to your child's preschool teacher about it. Then, if you are still "on the fence" about whether or not to start your son in kindergarten this year, a testing evaluation that includes a look at his cognitive skills, attention level, fine-motor skills, language skills, social abilities, and emotional maturity will likely give you helpful information about his readiness. Although the final decision is yours to make, the evaluator can assist you in weighing the pros and cons of starting now versus waiting another year.

Q: My daughter's third-grade teacher told me that he has recommended that she get a team evaluation. He said he is concerned about her math skills and wants to see if she has a learning problem. Should I go through with this?

A: It is a good sign that your daughter's teacher is paying attention to her learning and skill level. His recommendation for a team evaluation, which is described in detail in the next chapter, suggests that she is lagging behind her peers in her ability to understand or retain the math concepts he is teaching in class or in her ability to perform mental calculations. It is your legal right to accept or refuse his recommendation, but we suggest that you follow up on his concerns one way or another. That is, either have your daughter undergo the team evaluation at school or seek outside testing with a private clinician qualified to do to the testing (see Chapter Three). The next chapter reviews the advantages and disadvantages of both types of evaluations to help you make an informed choice.

A *private clinician* is a trained, licensed professional who works outside of the school system in a hospital, clinic, or agency.

Behavior

Perhaps there is no broader category than behavior, but in this section we focus on the main issues that we see in a clinical setting. That is, the concerns that are included here are significant enough to warrant seeking "professional help" and are typically not part of normal development. Though many kids will show these behaviors at various times, it's usually the severity and duration that make the behavior a true problem.

It is important to note that usually a problematic behavior is a sign that *something else is wrong*. Zach, our first grader who couldn't sit still for Circle Time in preschool and now is having trouble staying seated long enough to learn, is not simply a brat who has decided he'd rather move around than participate in class. Indeed, the "something else wrong" turned out to be attention-deficit/hyperactivity disorder (ADHD), a neurologically based learning disability that causes some children to be excessively active. Nicole, the teenager whose grades and mood went downhill during her freshman year of high school, might be clinically depressed, have an undiagnosed learning disability, or both; as her mother intuited, Nicole was *not* simply "being a teenager," as her behavior might have suggested to someone less savvy. So, with these things in mind, take a look at the following list and consider whether or not any of these concerns apply to your child:

Preschool and Up

- Has frequent explosive tantrums beyond age three
- Exhibits overly aggressive or destructive behavior
- Is excessively moody or irritable (yes, even in your teenager, this is not necessarily normal)
- Performs repetitive behaviors such as handwashing or checking
- Insists on having things a certain way or strictly following a routine
- Uses fantasy play excessively or daydreams

- Has frequent nightmares or sleeping difficulties
- Reacts strongly or not strongly enough to touch, pain, sound, and other types of stimulation
- Displays general fearfulness and frequent worrying
- Loses interest in friends or activities
- Suffers self-inflicted cuts, usually on arms and legs
- Is overly preoccupied with weight/dieting/exercising
- Loses or gains 10 percent or more of her original body weight
- Demonstrates impulsive or unsafe behavior
- Chooses friends who are "high risk" (e.g., may smoke, break the law, do drugs)
- Has odd ideas or preoccupations
- Reports seeing or hearing things that are not there (usually in a child over age six)
- Hoards food or steals compulsively
- Lies or cheats excessively
- Plays with fire or sets fires
- Demonstrates frequent sexualized play or talk
- Is socially isolated or withdrawn from others
- Skips school or refuses to attend
- Has poor hygiene/grooming habits at school age or adolescence
- Verbalizes a wish to die or kill himself

Though there is great variability in the kinds of problems described here, as well as in their root causes—such as depression, sensory integration dysfunction, trauma or abuse, or autism—typically your child will be referred by the pediatrician to a mental health professional such as a *child psychologist, child psychiatrist,* or *licensed social worker.* If it is determined that psychological testing is needed, only psychologists who have specialized training are capable of performing the appropriate testing evaluations for these concerns. At times the psychologist will determine whether a follow-up evaluation is needed, perhaps with a neurologist if a developmental disorder such as autism is diagnosed or with an occupational therapist if sensory integration dysfunction is suspected. In Chapter Three we discuss the different types of professionals whom you may come across in the process of getting your child the right kind of help, so you'll understand all this lingo in no time.

Q: *My husband and I are going through a divorce, and I'm concerned about the effect this might be having on my children. My twelve-year-old daughter won't talk about it and acts as if nothing is wrong, but I hear her crying at night. She is also suddenly afraid to play outside with friends and has started to turn down invitations to parties and other activities. Even though I keep trying, she refuses to open up to me. What should I do?*

A: It sounds as if you're right to be concerned. Divorce affects many children each year, but they often deal with it in different ways. Because your daughter isn't talking to you about her feelings and appears to be pulling back from her friends, it would probably be a good idea to seek professional assistance in providing support and intervention for her. If she still has trouble opening up to a child mental health professional, a psychological testing evaluation that includes projective testing may be helpful. These kinds of tests allow a sort of window into your child's inner world and may shed some light on how she is feeling. Is she feeling guilty? Angry? Confused? Why? Is she depressed or suffering from anxiety? If so, what kind of intervention would be best for her? These questions may be answered with the help of a good testing evaluation.

Making the Decision

We assume that if you've picked up this book you have some sense that your child is experiencing difficulty in some aspect of life and that you want to help. Without making it seem as though testing evaluations can answer every question about your child's development and well-being, we want to emphasize its many uses and roles.

The different types of testing evaluations, which are described in more detail later in the book, can tell you your child's general developmental level in language, motor, social, behavioral, and emotional functioning. Testing can provide an estimate of your child's innate ability, often referred to as *intelligence level,* and assess her cognitive strengths and weaknesses. A comprehensive evaluation with the right evaluator should give you information about your child's academic skills, too, such as the grade level of his reading skills or where she is relative to her peers in math or writing. Testing may also give you information about your child's various processing skills—how she takes in information from the world through her different senses and how she is able to use that information. For the purposes of making diagnoses, documenting the need for therapies or services, and figuring out the potential basis of an

> **Cognitive** skills or functioning relate to a person's capacity for perception, memory, attention, reasoning, and judgment.

emotional or behavioral problem, testing evaluations are typically essential.

When is testing not useful? There are certainly some questions that a testing evaluation can't answer. For example, no evaluation, even with the most experienced clinician, should predict your child's future long-term functioning. We have worked with families who were told by professionals that their children would never talk or could not learn to read (and they were wrong). No human being is capable of knowing the full potential of another person or the extent to which that person may benefit from interventions. These evaluations can give you a sense of what your child's current limitations may be and may estimate what kinds of problems your child could encounter down the road. However, the main purpose of a testing evaluation is to come up with solutions to the problems by recommending the right kinds of supports and interventions.

Factors to Consider

The decision to seek a testing evaluation of any kind is important for a few reasons. First, the process is a rather time-consuming and potentially expensive (see Chapter Two for more information on this). Second, because testing evaluations should not be repeated too often, you want to make sure that you are having your child evaluated at the right time with the right professional for the job. You also need to be open to what the evaluation may find with respect to your child's level of need. If you are having trouble accepting the findings, you are not very likely to pursue the recommended treatments or services with much enthusiasm—and, often, it's the parents' level of investment and motivation that is key to getting their children the help they need.

Is It Just Me?

Sometimes only the parents are concerned enough about their child's problem to seek a testing evaluation. Zach's mom, despite the pediatrician's initial conclusion that his difficulties were simply due to immaturity, felt strongly that he needed to be evaluated. You should know that, regardless of who agrees with you about your concerns, *it is your right to seek an evaluation at any time.* If your child's pediatrician won't give you a referral or make a formal request for a testing evaluation to your insurance company, you may be stuck with more expense than if the doctor had supported your decision to pursue an evaluation. However, there are alternatives to having the testing evaluations done *privately*, or through insurance or self-payment. Chapter Two discusses every child's right to state and federal funding for almost all types of testing evaluations, in which case you pay nothing.

Q: *I have suspected that there has been something a little "off" with my son for years now, and I have to say it has caused me a great deal of stress, mainly because I haven't known how to help him. Do a lot of parents go through this?*

A: Yes! We've focused mainly on your child so far—what it is that may be different about your son or daughter that is causing you concern. But it's critical to acknowledge what it's like for you to start out with a lingering doubt or worry about your child and to end up with what might be full-fledged distress at times. This is one of the reasons we have written this book: We want you to know that tuning in to your child's needs and knowing that something should be done makes you an outstanding parent, and we want to give you the tools and knowledge you need to follow up on that instinct. Like the parents we introduced you to at the beginning of this chapter, you may feel quite worried about your child, fearing that he won't be able to finish school or hold down a job, wondering if these problems are occurring because you didn't read to him enough when he was little or because he was born prematurely. It's also common for people to mistakenly believe that smart kids can't have learning disabilities or that a happy family can't have a child with emotional or behavioral problems. Because they can and do, by the millions each year, it is important to learn about this often critical intervention in your child's life. The fears and confusion that often accompany having your child tested are the other main reasons for this book. We hope that in the chapters ahead you will find the answers that will help you understand your child's needs better and allow you to get him the help that every child deserves.

Even if you're not sure whether or not to seek a testing evaluation for your child, we encourage you to read ahead to see what the process is like and to get a few tips on how to make it go as well as possible for you and your child. In our many years of experience, it is a rare case in which a testing evaluation has not provided critical information about the child that in turn makes a major difference in his life.

Two

What Is Involved
in a Testing Evaluation?

Though Philip's parents had decided they wanted to have him tested for his school problems, they didn't know where to begin. Is testing something his teacher would do? Should they talk with their pediatrician first? Was the testing process going to be stressful or upsetting for Philip? Would their insurance pay for it? Was the testing expensive?

Maybe you, like Philip's parents, have decided to have your child tested for a suspected concern. We hope you've found some relief in having made the decision and in knowing that you're likely to get helpful information from the test results. As we discussed in Chapter One, it's a good idea to talk with your child's pediatrician about the concerns you have, because the doctor may help guide you in getting the right kind of evaluation with the best type of professional for the job. In most situations you'll have the option of getting the evaluation through public or private agencies. Public agencies would include federal- and state-funded programs such as Early Intervention (EI) and the public school system. Private sources would include clinicians who practice in settings such as hospitals, community clinics, and private practices. Many factors may affect your decision about where to obtain your child's evaluation, including the type of concerns that you have, the cost, whether or not your insurance will pay for the evaluation, and the availability of private agencies.

For concerns such as language development, motor skills, or social

The First Evaluation: Private or Public?
The Pros and Cons

Pros

Public	Private
• You pay nothing for the evaluation.	• Some insurance plans will cover the cost of the evaluation in full or in part.
• The person who does the testing will often be the one to work with your child if he needs help.	• Some tests cannot be repeated within a specific amount of time (e.g., one year); you may want the private clinician to have full access to all tests rather than being limited to those that the school's evaluator did not use.
• The services recommended by the school system or EI will usually be paid for or provided by them at no cost to you.	
• You have the right to seek amendments to the school's reports.	• You have more confidence that the recommendations are being made without regard to the cost of the services, education model(s) preferred by the school system, and so forth.
• If you are not satisfied with the school's testing or conclusions, you have the right to get an independent evaluation at the school's expense.	
	• You may request editing of personal information from the report.
	• You control who sees the report and may have input into what recommendations are made.
	• You choose the evaluator.
	• You can usually get a more comprehensive evaluation from a private evaluator.
	(*cont.*)

The First Evaluation: Private or Public? (cont.)	
Cons	
Public	**Private**
• You do not get to choose the evaluator. • The process of having your child evaluated through the school system often takes a long time (rarely less than two months from referral to team meeting/Individualized Education Plan). • You do not control the report; it becomes part of your child's record automatically. • Even if the school will pay for an independent evaluation after having completed their own evaluation, your child now has to go through the same process all over again, and the independent evaluator is somewhat limited in the tests she can use.	• Sometimes the school will not fully accept the private evaluation and insist on doing their own testing. • There is usually quite a wait for an appointment, often up to three to six months. • Many insurance plans will not cover the full cost of testing by not authorizing enough hours to do a complete evaluation or by denying payment for the service altogether.

skills in children under three years of age, it is often recommended that they be evaluated by the local Early Intervention program, which is a federally funded program available in all states for babies and children up until their third birthday. By seeking the testing evaluation services from EI, you will have the cost covered (you pay nothing), and the treatment team may already be familiar with your child should some type of therapy be recommended. Preschooler Alexandria was tested by the speech and language therapist through the area EI team when she was two and a half and was found to show delays in her ability to understand and express herself with language. She also displayed some social delays in that she did not seem as interactive and engaged as most children her age. As a result, she was seen weekly for speech and language therapy and social facilitation, both provided in her home by the EI team. The cost of these therapies was also covered fully under the EI program without regard to the family's income.

In most circumstances, for kids from age three through a cutoff age established by state law for special education services (usually age twenty-one or twenty-two), it would be appropriate to request testing through your public school system, even for concerns that do not necessarily seem school-related. Five-year-old Alan was having trouble using scissors, drawing, playing with small toys, and buttoning his coat. When Alan's parents spoke with his pediatrician, they learned that he might have fine-motor skill delays. They were surprised to find out that Alan could be seen by the appropriate clinician, an occupational therapist, through their public school system. After finding that he was indeed lagging in the development of these skills, the school provided Alan with weekly occupational therapy, even though he wasn't enrolled in public school yet. And the cost of the evaluation and treatment was covered by the state and U.S. governments through tax dollars and other sources of education funding.

But how did Alan's parents even come to know about what the school system could offer? Like Philip's parents and countless others,

---

Q: My seventeen-month-old son is still not walking, and I'm getting worried. I've heard that it's my right to have him evaluated by my town's Early Intervention program, but is that my only option?

A: No, it isn't. Although there are many advantages to having your son evaluated by the EI team in your area, such as free assessment and treatment if there is a need, some parents choose to have their child seen by a private clinician. If this is your preference, you should speak with your pediatrician about your concerns regarding your son's development and ask for a referral. The appropriate clinician for this will probably be a licensed pediatric physical therapist or a pediatric orthopedist. The cost for this type of evaluation is generally covered by insurance companies, but you may have to pay a portion of the cost, depending on your particular insurance plan and/or the professional you see. Usually, pediatricians have several names of professionals that they have worked with before, and they can direct you to their offices for appointments.

---

they knew only that there was a possible problem and had little information about how to address it. At the pediatrician's recommendation, Alan's parents contacted their school system's special education office. They told the director about their concerns, and she then mailed them a packet of information about what services the school system could provide, how to obtain these services, the legal rights they had as parents, and so on. To save you some time, we provide here some general information about getting an evaluation for your child through the public school system. (The following information is based on federal law; the laws of your state may provide you with additional rights. Make sure you get a copy of these from your school district.)

Getting the Evaluation through the Public School System

After talking with your child's pediatrician and teacher about your concerns, you may decide that you would like your child evaluated through the school system. This means that the entire cost of the evaluation is covered; there is no expense to you or your insurance company. Anyone is eligible for a public school–based evaluation, regardless of income or whether or not your child actually attends the public schools. That is, if your child is age three or older but not yet in school, she is still entitled to a fully funded evaluation through your public school system. And, if your child has been suspended or expelled from public school, he is still eligible for a full evaluation at the school system's expense. This also means that if your child is going to a private school, he is still eligible for any type of evaluation that the public school system can provide (see the sidebar "Public School Evaluation Options"). Nicole, who was in ninth grade at a private Catholic school in a neighboring town, received a full evaluation through her town's public school system for possible learning problems and/or depression. One of her teachers then attended the team meeting and served as a liaison between the private school and public school special education staff.

A **team meeting** consists of all of the participating school staff who have completed aspects of the evaluation and/or who would be responsible for helping the child if so recommended, in addition to the parents and child when appropriate.

The first step in obtaining your child's testing evaluation through the public school system is to make a referral, or request for testing, to the special education department for your school system. You should call the special education office for your school district with this request, and follow up the call with a letter stating your request for your child's evaluation *in writing*. Once the school gets your request for an evaluation, it should contact you. State law may require that the school district respond within a certain time frame; the period may vary from state to state.

Because you may not know what kind of evaluation your child might need, it is often best to request what may be termed a *pre-evaluation conference*. This is a meeting between you and at least one member of the special education team, usually the chairperson, to talk about your concerns. You will discuss what kind of testing will be helpful and who will be doing the evaluations at school. Though the specific types of evaluations may vary from child to child, *you should always request that a full intelligence measure be given to get an estimate of your child's potential*. Schools will not always perform intelligence testing, but it is essential for figuring out your child's areas of relative strength and weakness. Chapter Four has more information about this, but know that you will need a test such as the WISC-IV, the Stanford–Binet, or the Differential Abilities Scale (DAS) to give you needed information about your child's potential to learn and perform. If school personnel do not have the ability to perform such testing, the district can always send you to an outside evaluator at the school's expense.

A preevaluation conference usually provides more information and allows you to get to know at least one member of the special education staff before testing has started. With more information, you and your child are better prepared for what to expect; usually, the more you know up front, the more comfortable you will be with the process.

Getting the Ball Rolling

Regardless of whether you've had a preevaluation conference, the school district must send you advance written notice about the kinds of testing evaluations it plans to do with your child, as well as notice of the procedural safeguards available to you (e.g., your rights to reject testing, confidentiality of student records, etc.). Be aware that you have the right to consent to some evaluations but not others. For example, you may agree with the need to do a speech and language evaluation but not an occupational therapy evaluation. You may also request that additional evaluations be performed if the school's proposal does not cover all the areas in which you suspect your child has needs or concerns (see the sidebar "Public School Evaluation Options").

Q: *My twelve-year-old daughter is about to be tested at school for suspected learning problems. What should I tell her about it?*

A: We agree that it's a good idea to give your daughter some explanation about what will be taking place at school. She probably knows she's having some trouble with certain subjects or skills, so you can use this knowledge to help her understand why she's going to be getting some testing. For example, say she's having difficulty with reading—you could say something like, "You know how sometimes it's hard for you to do the reading homework you get? Well, I've talked with your teacher, and you'll be meeting with Mr. Jones and Ms. Thompson a few times over the next week or so to do some testing. This will help us find out how you learn best so we know how to make reading easier and more fun for you." You can reassure her that she will not miss too much class and that the tests do not count toward her school grades; they are intended just to help you figure out how she learns. If she has a lot of questions that you don't feel prepared to answer, you should feel free to have her meet with the school guidance counselor to talk more about what she can expect.

Once you agree with what the school proposes to provide in the evaluation of your child, *you must give written consent before the school will begin the evaluation.* Federal law states that the evaluation must be completed within a reasonable period of time after the school receives the parent's consent; the law of your state may specify a particular number of days within which the school must complete all necessary tests. The child must be assessed in all areas of suspected weakness or disability; thus, depending on the concerns that brought you to have your child tested, more than one type of evaluation may be needed. Often the school system will provide a multidisciplinary evaluation, which is a comprehensive assessment that usually includes several of the types of testing listed in the sidebar (see Chapter Four for specific test descriptions). All standardized tests must be administered by appropriately trained and knowledgeable personnel.

Special Education: Is Your Child Eligible?

The school-based evaluation should examine all areas of a suspected weakness or disability that significantly affect school performance. The best practice is for the school to provide a detailed description of your

Public School Evaluation Options

Intelligence testing: This gives an estimate of your child's potential for learning. All other test scores from the school's team evaluation should be compared with your child's estimated potential to find relative strengths and weaknesses. This then helps to determine the need for services from the school.

Educational/Achievement testing: This is testing in various subject areas such as reading, math, and writing to find the grade level of your child's skills.

Emotional/Behavioral testing (usually called "psychological testing" in private settings): A psychologist should perform this evaluation, which includes an assessment of your child's emotional, social, and behavioral functioning. This should include class observation, recess and lunchtime observation, parent and teacher rating scales, child self-report tests, and projective tests such as the Thematic Apperception Test (TAT), drawings, or sentence completion test.

Speech and Language testing: This evaluation assesses your child's ability to speak clearly, understand language, and express himself with language. Social communication skills called "pragmatics," which include eye contact, initiating social contact, turn taking in conversation, and gestures, should also be assessed.

Occupational Therapy testing: An occupational therapist will observe and evaluate your child's fine- and gross-motor skills, visual–spatial and visual–motor skills, sensory processing and integration skills, and general self-help skills.

Physical Therapy testing: This evaluation is usually necessary for assessing your child's balance, gross-motor coordination, muscle strength, and movement.

Home Assessments: An assessment of pertinent family history and home situation factors such as parental divorce, living arrangements, and the like is often done as part of the school district's evaluation. Home visits are sometimes made by a special education team member, and the child's complete developmental history is taken through parent interviews. Estimates of adaptive behavior at home, school, and in the community are also made using interviews and certain measures such as the Vineland Adaptive Behavior Scale.

Vision/Hearing/General Health Assessments: Though most pediatricians will perform these evaluations, the school system is available to perform vision screens, hearing tests, and physicals for children.

child's needs in a written report that gives all test scores, observations, findings, conclusions, and, most important, recommendations for treatment or services. (State law may provide specific requirements for the form and content of an evaluation report.)

Disability refers to an area of weakness substantial enough to warrant some type of service or intervention.

The evaluation process is designed to help the evaluation team answer two questions to determine whether by law your child is eligible for school-funded special education services. (Make sure you refer to your state law for additional information about how it defines the need for special education services.)

1. Does the child have a disability? What type? (See the sidebar "Disability Types under Special Education Law [IDEA].")
2. Does the child, by reason of his disability, need specially designed instruction and related services (e.g., speech and language therapy)?

For your child to be found eligible for special education, the answer to both of these questions must be yes. The Individuals with Disabilities Education Act (IDEA) is the federal law that defines a child's right to special education and related services; each state law can provide additional rights to children but cannot go below the level of protection set forth in IDEA. So, regardless of what state you live in, your child will be eligible for school-funded special education services if he falls into one or more of the disability categories specified in IDEA (summarized in the sidebar). Again, check your state law, because there may be additional disability categories that allow your child to receive special education services.

The Evaluation Meeting

How does the school system determine whether or not your child qualifies for special education? The school evaluation is the first step. After the testing is completed, the school will call a meeting to discuss the evaluation results and recommendations (state law may specify an amount of time within which the meeting must be held). Parents must receive notice of the meeting far enough in advance to ensure that they will be able to attend. The notice must specify who will be coming to

Disability Types under Special Education Law (IDEA)

To be categorized as a child with a disability under IDEA, the child must have one or more of the following impairments, and the impairment must adversely affect her educational performance:

- Specific learning disability (e.g., a significant delay in reading, math, or writing not attributable to another disability such as mental retardation)
- Autism
- Mental retardation
- Emotional disturbance, meaning a condition such as depression or anxiety that exists over a long period of time or to a marked degree
- Speech and language impairment, meaning a communication disorder (e.g., stuttering, impaired articulation, expressive or receptive language deficits, etc.)
- Traumatic brain injury, meaning an acquired injury to the brain caused by an external physical force (including birth trauma) that results in a functional disability or psychosocial impairment
- Severe orthopedic impairment, such as cerebral palsy, amputation, etc.
- "Other Health Impairment" (e.g., attention-deficit disorders, asthma, diabetes, heart condition, etc.)
- Sensory impairment such as in hearing and/or vision
- (In many states: developmental delays in communication, physical abilities, cognition, social/emotional skills, or adaptive skills for children ages three to nine)

the meeting. If the proposed meeting date, time, or place is not convenient, parents and the school district must find a mutually agreeable alternative.

You should request copies of the evaluation reports in advance of the meeting. *You must ask the school for copies of these reports,* because typically you will not automatically get them in advance. It is important for you to go over the reports before the meeting, to discuss them with others who are knowledgeable about your child, and to come up with a list of questions to ask. Chapters 4 and 5 will help you in understanding the numbers and terms often used in these reports. At the meeting, the members of the evaluation team should also explain their findings and how the recommendations will be helpful to your child.

Each evaluation team meeting must include the parents or legal guardians; at least one regular education teacher; a special education teacher or provider if your child is already getting such services (e.g., if your child is turning three and has been receiving EI); a staff person from the school district who knows the resources in the system and who is qualified to provide or supervise special education services; a school staff person who can interpret the evaluation results with respect to how the child will be serviced and instructed in school (often, this is someone previously listed); and, if appropriate, the child. Note that the child must be invited to attend the meeting once she is fourteen or older but does not have to go.

Parents or the school district can bring others to the meeting with them. If your child is seeing a therapist in the community, for example, it may be helpful for this professional to come to the meeting. She may be able to clarify certain findings and can get information that will be useful to her in treating your child. It is wise to inform the school in advance if you plan to bring anyone with you to the meeting who was not listed as an attendee on its notice of the meeting.

Input from you (and in many instances from your child as well) is essential to making the meeting and the resulting education changes as effective as possible. Before the evaluation meeting, we encourage you to talk with your child about what she wants from her education. What would she like help with? What would he change if he could? What are her goals for herself? This discussion should include hopes and dreams, big and little; don't feel constrained by reality. If your daughter says she hopes to learn what she needs to know to be president of the United States, then that's OK. If she wants help organizing her backpack, that's OK, too. Your vision (and your child's) should help guide the team in developing an education program that will move the child toward her goals, no matter how big or small they may be.

The primary decision made at the evaluation meeting is whether or not your child is eligible for special education services. Generally speaking, the IDEA states that any child may be eligible for services if he suffers from one of the listed disabilities in the preceding sidebar and if the disability has an adverse effect on his educational performance. For many of the disability categories, though not all, it is necessary to consider whether there is a significant difference between the child's ability (usually measured with intelligence tests) and performance (e.g., reading level, math level, language skills, handwriting, coordination skills, social skills).

Fourth grader Philip, for example, was found to have a high-average level of intelligence but was reading at the second-grade level. Because a severe discrepancy appeared between his intellectual ability and his reading level that could not be explained by any other factor, and because the deficit could be remedied by specially designed instruction, Philip was found eligible for special education under the specific-learning-disability category.

The Individualized Education Plan

When a student is found to be eligible for special education services, a document called an *Individualized Education Plan*, or an *IEP*, is developed at the evaluation meeting and/or at a separate, later meeting using the evaluation results. Federal law specifies that the meeting to develop the IEP must be held within thirty days of the time the child is found eligible for special education services; state law may impose a shorter deadline. State law may also specify the amount of time within which the school must provide you with the proposed IEP document.

Once you receive the IEP from the school, you may accept or reject it, in whole or in part. If you agree that the IEP accurately discusses your child's needs and provides the services and modifications necessary to help the child, then you should sign the IEP and return it to the designated person immediately, as it is in your child's best interests to do so. Unless the IEP indicates a different start date, *all of the changes stated in the IEP must be implemented immediately.* We urge you to check on this within a week or two of signing the IEP, as we have heard about children who waited many months to start their services or who do not receive the services as often as the IEP states they will. Although school staff members want to help your child, sometimes a shortage of resources or scheduling conflicts will prevent them from fulfilling the IEP services right away. These are not valid reasons to deny or delay services specified in the IEP, however. You will need to be a strong advocate for your child, because there should be no excuses for not giving her what she is entitled to by law. In fact, you have the right to receive *compensatory services* at the school's expense should you find that they have not been providing services as stated in the IEP that you signed. Tina's parents were able to get the school system to pay for private speech and language therapy sessions twice a week for six months to make up for the time the school did not provide her with this service, which was specified in her IEP.

If you think that only certain aspects of the IEP are appropriate for your child, you can partially accept the IEP. Or, if you find the entire IEP unacceptable in that the services or modifications listed are not a good fit or frequent enough for your child's needs, you will want to reject it. Whether you accept the IEP in its entirety, select only portions of it, or reject it altogether, your IEP response should be given in writing; that is, you should write a brief letter to the school district clearly stating that you accept all the terms of the IEP or some of the terms of the IEP (and write down which ones you reject) or that you reject the entire IEP. State law may specify the amount of time you have to respond to the school, so make sure you check on this.

Once you accept the IEP (or the accepted portion, if you accept only part), it becomes a legally binding contract between you as the parent and the school as to what services your child will receive. Therefore, you should review the IEP carefully before responding, and we encourage you to have other relevant people look it over as well. Your child's pediatrician, special education advocate (see the discussion of educational advocates later in this chapter), or therapist, for example, may be helpful to you in deciding whether what the school has offered to provide is enough to meet your child's needs. *All the services and accommodations listed in the child's IEP are delivered at no cost to the family,* so you don't need to worry about covering the expense of whatever therapies and specialized instruction the school is recommending. You should also know that, if the school system cannot provide a recommended service for your child, the school will pay for an outside provider to work with your child and/or pay to transport your child to another school, where she can receive the appropriate services at the school's expense.

It's important for you to know that an IEP is not a newly designed curriculum for your child. Rather, it provides services and accommodations that will help your child participate and progress in the *general curriculum,* the curriculum that other students his age without disabilities are learning. This is mandated by the IDEA. For some kids, an IEP will include changes in *methodology* (how the curriculum is taught) so as to best meet their needs. Philip, who was found to have a reading disability (a specific learning disability), was offered small-group reading instruction separate from his regular class; three times a week, he and

Q: I've looked over my daughter's IEP many times, but as I'm not an educator, I don't know if what the school has recommended for her is enough. How can I be sure?

A: This is a common question among parents. After all, how are you supposed to know how often your child should meet with the speech and language therapist or whether once or twice a week is better for social skills training? You're welcome to call the school contact person, usually the IEP team chairperson, to ask questions about the IEP. As we mentioned before, you should feel free to ask your child's pediatrician or another relevant person in your child's life to review the IEP. If you are still unsure and you don't mind the expense, you can hire an education consultant or a specialist in the area of concern to review the school's reports and the IEP to figure out if it's appropriate.

two other students went to the resource room to work with the reading specialist for forty-five-minute sessions.

An IEP may also include modifications in the content of the curriculum so that the information is made less complex for the student. It may list accommodations that generally allow the child to remain in the regular classroom with adjustments to address his disability. For example, Isabelle was found to have an auditory processing disorder and, as a result, has trouble learning from class lectures. She was given visual aids and a written outline of the lesson so that she could improve her understanding of what is being discussed in class. Thomas, who was found eligible for special education due to a birth defect to his hand, had such impaired handwriting that he received the accommodation in his IEP of being able to dictate his answers to test questions.

As we all know, children may need help in areas other than academics. The IEP is also intended to address these types of concerns. The IDEA requires the IEP to contain a statement about the child's present levels of educational performance, including the ways in which the disability affects his involvement or progress in the general curriculum (including recess, gym class, etc.). For preschoolers, this statement would include how the disability affects the child's participation in appropriate activities (Circle Time, playtime). The IEP must discuss and address not only the child's academic needs but also all other educational needs that result from her disability. This may mean that the IEP includes modifications and services such as social skills training, picture communication systems for language-impaired children, behavioral management, and assistance during gym class. You and the team members should be as creative and resourceful as possible to come up with strategies for helping your child in school.

How Will We Know It's Helping?

For each area of need resulting from the child's disability, the IEP must contain a measurable annual goal. These goals should show the expected progress or growth your child will make over the next year of receiving services. For example, one of Philip's goals was "Philip will be able to read grade-level text and answer questions about what he has read with at least 80 percent accuracy." One of Alexandria's goals in her IEP was "Alexandria will make improved eye contact with the person who is speaking to her." The information under each goal must include benchmarks, or short-term objectives, such as "Philip will improve his ability to decode two-syllable words." The IEP must also state how the child's progress toward the annual goals will be measured and by whom and how the parents will be informed of the child's progress.

A key section of the IEP describes the special education, related services (such as occupational therapy), and modifications to be provided to the child. Here the school system states clearly, often in chart form, what services will be provided to your child, how often (frequency and duration), and by whom. This section should also specify the location (e.g., whether your child will be pulled out for services or receive them in the classroom).

The term **pulled out** refers to having the child leave his primary classroom to receive the given service elsewhere, such as the resource room or special education class, as opposed to having the specialist come into the class to provide the specialized instruction.

If you are concerned about your child having a three-month break from services over the summer, *extended school year services* are often recommended. This typically means that the services (which may be the same as or different from those provided during the school year, depending on the needs of the child) will be given to your child for at least a portion of the summer vacation. If the services will be different over the summer, however, the IEP must state what the changes will be. Carl, who is autistic, was given speech and language therapy, occupational therapy, and social skills training at a school-based special-needs camp for most of the summer. As these were included on his IEP, the cost for these interventions was covered entirely by the school system.

Sometimes the public school system cannot meet the needs of certain children, and an alternative placement is recommended. This means that another school program, such as a private school for learning-disabled students, a residential school, or a therapeutic day school, may be necessary. It was clear to the school's evaluation team that Victor, for example, needed a residential school, after he had many violent outbursts at school and home. IDEA states that the child must be placed in "the least restrictive environment" that will meet his needs; that is, the parents and the public school system need to find a placement for him that meets but does not exceed the level of supervision he needs. The cost of an alternative placement and transportation to it is covered by the public school when it has been recommended by the evaluation team and stated in the student's IEP.

A **residential school** is an alternative placement that provides the child with twenty-four-hour supervision, as well as educational, behavioral, and social training. As the name implies, the students live at the school but may be able to go home on weekends or during vacations. A **therapeutic day school** is usually appropriate for students who are unable to attend public school due to major mental illness or behavioral disturbance. It is considered less restrictive than a residential school, and the students go home after school and on weekends, for vacations, and at other times when school is not in session.

Having said all this, we need to acknowledge what is referred to as the *FAPE standard*. *FAPE* stands for "free and appropriate education," meaning that, although each child is not guaranteed the absolute best in education and other resources, the services must be appropriate given the child's needs and must allow her to make educational progress. So, even if your area has an outstanding private school for children with learning disabilities, the public school system does not have to pay for your child to go there if it is able to give her enough services to help her make adequate progress. However, if you can document that, despite the public school's best efforts, your child is not making educational progress, you may be able to get the school system to fund your child's placement at such a private school. Be aware that obtaining such funding usually requires at least a school year's worth of failure on your child's part and typically a battle with the school system, as these placements can cost $20,000 to $40,000 a year a more.

Section 504 Plan

Q: I just came from my daughter's evaluation team meeting, and I am feeling really frustrated. I know she has a problem understanding what she reads, but the school evaluation showed she is performing only a few months below grade level. She came out with an average intelligence level, so they said her scores don't show any learning problems. I know she needs some help, though; what can I do?

A: Your daughter is in good company. Many kids fall into the gray area of learning weaknesses, in which a formal disability cannot be supported by the school's results but problems still clearly exist.

If the evaluation team agrees that the child has a disability but does not believe that it is significant enough to require special education, then the team should consider whether the child would benefit from accommodations or services under a *Section 504 Plan.* Section 504 of the Rehabilitation Act of 1973 applies to students who have learning or performance weaknesses that could be deemed "disabilities" but that are not eligible for special education. Such a child may have an academic program or curriculum modified to meet her needs or may receive accommodations such as extra time when taking tests. Accommodations or services such as this should be written into a Section 504 Plan, which is similar in concept to an IEP but is usually less detailed and not considered "special education." It is important to note that fewer parental legal rights are associated with a 504 Plan. For example, a 504 Plan for a child can be discontinued without a formal meeting with the parents, whereas an IEP cannot be "dropped" without proving that the child has met his goals and that there is no further need for the services.

The Section 504 accommodation plan can vary a lot in what it can provide a student. Often children who have attention-deficit/hyperactivity disorder (ADHD) but no other learning problems cam have their needs met with a Section 504 Plan. Accommodations such as preferential seating, organization skills support, testing in isolation, and breaking tasks up into smaller sections will be specified in a 504 Plan for such kids. Depending on the needs of the child, such measures may give enough support for them to learn at an expected level. It should be noted that in some states a related service, such as speech and language therapy, may be placed under a Section 504 Plan, as the need for only this type of intervention may not qualify the child for special education or an IEP.

If You and the School Don't Agree: Your Rights and Options

But what happens when you review the IEP or the 504 Plan and decide that it is *not* good enough to meet your child's needs? You have the option of rejecting the IEP or 504 Plan in whole or in part. When you do so, you put all the services recommended by the school on hold; your child continues in school just as he has been. You can reject only portions of either document, listing the areas of concern and then signing the form. The sections of the IEP or 504 Plan that you accepted will then be put into place immediately while you and the evaluation team try to come up with a new agreement. Or you can reject the entire proposed IEP or 504 Plan as inappropriate for meeting your child's needs but accept the provision of the services on an interim basis while you attempt to resolve the dispute. Either way, you should request a new team meeting to go over your concerns and to try to develop a more satisfactory program for your child. If you are able to do so, the school will mail out to you a revised IEP or Section 504 Plan for your response.

Following is a list of steps to take when you and the rest of the team don't agree on the findings or recommendations.

1. If an IEP or a Section 504 has been proposed but you don't accept some or all of it, put your response, including your concerns, in writing and request another team meeting to come up with a new IEP or 504 Plan.
2. If your child is not found eligible for an IEP or a 504 Plan but you feel he has some type of disability, request an independent educational evaluation (IEE) at the school's expense. Also, if you have tried step 1 and still can't agree, an IEE would be a good next move.
3. If the school appeals your request for an IEE, see if you can pay for an independent evaluation through your insurance or out of pocket.
4. If after obtaining an independent evaluation (either an IEE or one at your own expense), you and the school district cannot agree on what your child needs, voluntary mediation is recommended.
5. If mediation fails, you can pursue a hearing, but you will likely need a lawyer, and it will be time-consuming. You will need to figure out if this would cause more financial and emotional stress on you than would simply paying for private tutoring or

therapies. Sometimes, though, you may have no choice but to go to hearing, as in the case of a child who may need a residential program or a therapeutic school.

If you can't resolve your dispute with the school system informally, there are formal procedures available to you. Each state is required to ensure that parents and school districts are able to seek *voluntary mediation* and an *impartial due process hearing*. Through a state-designated agency, parents and schools can receive free mediation support to resolve disputes fairly quickly. As indicated by its name, the mediation is voluntary, meaning that both the school district and parents must agree to participate.

The designated agency also has the authority to hold formal hearings before an impartial hearing officer, who can decide any dispute relating to the identification, evaluation, or educational placement of a child with a disability. These hearings also serve to uphold the FAPE standard discussed previously. In other words, the officer decides whether or not the school system is providing appropriate educational services for the child given his needs.

Either you or the school district can request the hearing process; the parties may use the hearing office instead of or in addition to the mediation services.

The hearing is typically a last resort, as it can be expensive if you hire a lawyer (which is usually wise because the school district will have one) and quite time-consuming. The hearing officer's decision is legally binding and is final unless appealed. Some states have another level of administrative review, and others don't; either way, if you or the school district is not satisfied with the hearing decision, you have the right to appeal to federal district court or to an appropriate state court. If a hearing officer agrees with you that a change of placement is appropriate (e.g., a residential school), the school district must move your child to the new placement during the appeal process. If the hearing officer decides against you in a case such as this, the child remains in his current education setting during the appeals process unless you and the school agree otherwise.

Getting a Private Evaluation

In some cases parents opt to start with a private evaluation, for a variety of reasons laid out in the first sidebar in this chapter. A private evaluation allows you control over the report, and you may have more input as to the specific recommendations for your child, for example. You may also be aware that school systems often will not formally diagnose disorders such as dyslexia, autism, attention-deficit/hyperactivity disorder (ADHD), or a nonverbal learning disorder, though their results may clearly indicate that these diagnoses apply. If you are seeking a diagnosis and related recommendations for school and home, then a private evaluation is likely the best course of action for your child.

In the community, you will find psychologists, speech and language therapists, occupational therapists, and physical therapists, working in hospitals, clinics, and private practices, who will do their own evaluations with your child to figure out whether any areas of concern need to be addressed. To request the right type of evaluation for your child, though, you will need to have done some research. Unlike in the school system, in which the school determines what evaluations are appropriate for your child with your input, you need to know what to ask for when seeking a private evaluation.

So how do you know? A good place to start would be with your child's pediatrician. More and more, physicians are being trained in medical school or residency to know about the different types of testing evaluations available and how to tell when a child needs what kind of evaluation. Zach's pediatrician was concerned that he may have ADHD but did not want to prescribe medication without further assessment. He recommended to Zach's parents that he receive a neuropsychological evaluation to help figure out whether this diagnosis was accurate and what they could do for him at school and home to help him do his best. When the parents agreed, Zach's doctor gave them some names of a few licensed psychologists whom he had worked with before in similar situations. He asked Zach's parents to call each one to see who was available to see their son, to schedule an appointment, and then to let his office know who the evaluating psychologist would be. Zach's doctor would then call in a referral, or request for testing, to the family's insurance company to get authorization.

An *authorization* for a testing evaluation (like an authorization for certain medical procedures) means that your insurance company agrees to pay for a stated amount of time, often listed as "units," for a given evaluation. You need to check to see if the amount authorized will be enough to cover the full cost of the evaluation; if not, you will need to ask what your share of the expense will be.

Q: My wife and I have rejected most of our son's IEP, mainly because we don't think the evaluations done by the school were thorough enough to get at the problems we think are there. The team chairperson suggested that we obtain something called "an independent educational evaluation." What's that and how can it help us?

A: You've raised a very important issue—you can't have a good IEP without thorough evaluations that really portray the child's strengths and weaknesses. Federal law allows parents to get an *independent educational evaluation*, or *IEE*, at public expense if they disagree with an evaluation performed or obtained by the school district (the law in your state may provide you with additional rights—check it out). An IEE may cover an area of need already evaluated by the school district or an area that the school's evaluation failed to consider. The IEE is given to your child by a private clinician, someone not affiliated with or chosen by the school system. The examiner must be qualified to perform the evaluation, but the school district may not impose qualification requirements that are more stringent than those it uses in performing its own evaluations. The IEE must be provided at no cost to you. If the school system disagrees with the need for an IEE, it must initiate a due process hearing to prove that its evaluation was appropriate.

Of course, you have the right to obtain an independent evaluation at your own expense at any time. If you or your insurance pays for the independent evaluation, you may choose any professional. There is no need to inform the school district in advance of the evaluation, though if there is any question about the evaluator's credentials, it may be wise to run your choice by the school department to make sure they can't later claim that your professional wasn't qualified. Another advantage, if you are able to pay for the evaluation yourself or with your insurance, is that you control the results. You do not have to share the report with the school system, though usually you will want to; when you do, it becomes part of your child's school record. If the school pays for an IEE, by contrast, the school receives the results along with you and enters them into your child's record (though there is a procedure to dispute this through IDEA and the Right to Privacy Act).

Regardless of who pays, the evaluation/IEP team must consider the results of an independent evaluation. This does not mean that they must implement all of the recommended services from the independent evaluation, but they should hold a meeting with you and the other team members to discuss and respond to the new information. If the law in your state does not require the team to reconvene when a new evaluation report is presented, you should request that the team do so.

Q: After all that testing at school, we just received a letter stating that our daughter "is not eligible for special education services" and that nothing has been recommended for her. We can't believe it! What can we do now to help our daughter?

A: This is another situation in which an IEE may be helpful. Sometimes the school evaluations do not assess certain skills adequately or at all, such as attention, memory, processing, and organization. At other times, the school reports may conclude that there is not a problem even though you and your child know that something isn't as it should be. The independent evaluation can shed new light on the controversy, often clarifying the child's needs and providing recommendations for school-based and/or private services that will help your child succeed. Ultimately, if you can't reach an agreement with your school district, you will need to resort to mediation or a hearing to resolve the eligibility issue.

Q: My seven-year-old son just went through all the evaluations at school, and now he has to do more testing with an outside psychologist for an independent evaluation. How do I explain that to him?

A: Though it seems like a real burden on your child, ultimately it is really worth the extra effort needed to get an independent evaluation. And, for the most part, testing can be fun and different. Because many measures can't be repeated within a year, the independent evaluator will be using some similar, but not identical, tests with your son (as noted in our list of pros and cons at the beginning of this chapter, this is sometimes a good enough reason to have the independent evaluation done first, at your or your insurance company's expense). You can tell him that the reason he is meeting with Dr. Thomas is that you need to know more about how he learns so that school can go as well as possible for him. You can add that the school's evaluations did not find all the answers needed to help him best, so Dr. Thomas is going to help find these out. You may want to reward your son for all his hard work with a special treat, such as an ice cream cone or a new book, after the IEE appointment.

Q: *I'm worried that even with the results of my daughter's independent evaluation, which showed that she has a learning disability, the school system won't give her the services recommended. I feel that I need some help advocating for her needs–will the independent evaluator do that for her?*

A: Sometimes, but often you will need to pay him to do so, because this service is not typically included in the cost of the testing evaluation. Often, the evaluator's schedule doesn't allow him or her to attend school meetings very easily. Fortunately, there is a professional called an *educational advocate* whom you may hire for this purpose. These individuals are not lawyers but are usually quite knowledgeable about education law and know how to get the system to respond to your child's needs. They attend the team meetings and represent the results in the independent evaluation, usually after talking with the independent evaluator. They will sometimes confer with the evaluator after the meetings to talk about any ideas or changes that were discussed. You will usually not be charged for the time that the independent evaluator spends talking with your child's advocate, as most professionals consider this contact part of their responsibility in completing the evaluation process for your child.

Q: *What if we don't want to have our child tested through the schools but would like the school system to use the results of a private evaluation? Can we do that?*

A: Sometimes. We have seen some school systems welcome outside, or private, evaluations and use the results to develop a child's IEP or Section 504 Plan. Then again, we've worked with other kids whose schools said they would have to do their own evaluation before considering them for special education despite a perfectly good recent private evaluation. The school system has the right to insist on doing its own evaluation, but of course it takes more of their time, not to mention more energy from your child. It's probably a good idea to talk with your school's special education director before you have your child evaluated privately to see if the school is open to using the report from the private evaluation to figure out whether your child is eligible for services. If they say up front that they will have to do their own testing regardless of what the private evaluation shows, then you need to decide whether to forgo or postpone the private evaluation and start with the school's testing.

The Insurance Game

More and more, insurance companies are cutting back on what they will pay for testing evaluations, if anything at all. We are as perplexed as you are about this, especially because there is strong evidence that every kind of learning and emotional disability is at least in part biologically based. It usually helps if the referring doctor can make a case that the testing should be considered "medical" in nature. For example, rather than saying that Zach was having "school problems," his pediatrician said, "My patient is presenting with variable attention, trouble with memory, and difficulty with impulse control—I am requesting neuropsychological testing to rule out an organic/medical cause for these concerns and to arrive at an appropriate diagnosis." As soon as most insurance companies hear "school problems" or "learning problems," they immediately relegate the testing to the school system, assuming this is something that the school district can evaluate. Because of this, you will likely not receive authorization for the private evaluation. Therefore we advise you to talk about this concern with the referring doctor to arrive at honest ways of explaining the need for testing that are not just school related so as to increase the chances that this service will be covered.

Likewise, if you are concerned about your child's emotional well-being, we suggest that the referring clinician use formal psychiatric diagnoses as "rule outs" when making the referral for psychological testing. When nine-year-old Sandra was acting moody, nervous, irritable, and tired, her parents became concerned. So, when her pediatrician called in her request for testing authorization, she said, "I am requesting a full psychological evaluation to rule out major depression and generalized anxiety disorder." This was much more helpful than saying something like, "My patient seems sad and worried, so I would like psychological testing done."

Even when you and your referring doctor take these steps to improve the chances that the evaluation cost will be covered by your insurance company, there is no guarantee. You should know that you always have the right to appeal the authorization denial from your insurance company; the company should explain to you the proper course of action to take in order to do so. Sometimes the insurance company needs additional information from a therapist, a neurologist, or the like to support the need for testing. They may want to review the testing already done by the school (if this is an independent evaluation) to determine if any more testing is necessary. You don't have to give this information, but you should know that it is unlikely that they will change their decision to deny coverage without it.

Q: *My friend recommended a psychologist who saw her son for testing. She raved about her and said she was "the best." The problem is that this psychologist is not a covered provider for my insurance company. Is it worth paying more to see someone I've heard is really good, or are they all basically the same?*

A: Just like cars and washing machines, not all professionals are created equal. This goes for psychologists, speech and language therapists, occupational therapists, and the like. Word-of-mouth recommendations from friends or relatives are often helpful, especially as these sources usually know your child to some extent and may be familiar with the concerns that you have. If you're using an educational advocate, he is also likely to have suggestions. You may feel torn between going with someone on your provider list to do the evaluation and paying for part or all of the evaluation with the professional recommended to you by your friend. However, you should consider the benefits to your child of having a thorough evaluation with someone who will "go to bat" for your child if needed rather than gambling on something this important. To reduce your risk of getting an inadequate evaluation, you should read Chapter Three for the things to look for and to ask the clinician prior to making an appointment.

Q: *We've decided to have our daughter evaluated privately in a group practice that doesn't accept insurance. This means we will have to pay out of pocket for the whole thing. How much can we expect to be charged? What does the cost of the evaluation actually cover?*

A: Though the cost of an evaluation varies greatly depending on what kind of evaluation your daughter needs, where you live regionally, and who the professional is, we can give you some rough estimates here based on figures from the Northeast. For a full neuropsychological testing evaluation, which generally includes an intake (parent interview and/or forms), a review of any records, contact with the school or any other relevant sources, testing appointment(s) with the child ranging from two to five hours, test scoring, test interpretation, report writing, and a feedback meeting with the parents and/or child, the cost, as of early 2004, is typically in the range of $1,200 to $2,500. For a full psychological testing evaluation, the process is pretty much the same, but the testing time with the child is less, usually from one to two hours. The cost of this type of evaluation is usually around $500 to $800. For a full speech and language evaluation, you will likely pay somewhere around $700, though you could get a screening for about $250. A complete occupational therapy evaluation, including sensory processing, will probably cost around $1,000; a screening will be about the same cost as a speech and language

A **feedback meeting** allows you and the evaluator to go over the results of the evaluation together. You will often receive the report in advance so that you can review it and come up with questions before the feedback meeting.

screen—$250 or so. You should always receive a full written report from any type of evaluation that your child receives. The report should include the reason your child was seen, behavior observations, test results (including all test scores), a summary, and recommendations. For more information on understanding reports, see Chapter Five.

If you have to pay directly for any evaluation because the practice won't accept your insurance, make sure that you get a receipt from the evaluator with appropriate diagnostic codes, service codes, and tax identification number to submit to your insurance company. You may be able to get reimbursed for all or at least some of the cost of the evaluation. If nothing else, save the receipt to claim as a medical expense for that year.

Q: Our insurance company will not cover the cost of our son's evaluation, but we know he has to have it. The problem is, we simply can't afford to pay for it all at once. Is there such a thing as charging the expense to a credit card or paying the hospital or provider in monthly installments?

A: Almost always. Most hospitals these days are able to accept major credit cards for payment or offer monthly payment plans that can be arranged through the patient credit office. You should first check to see if you qualify for free care in the hospital where your child will be seen. They may also offer a sliding scale based on your annual family income. Many professionals in private practice also have sliding scales and can make arrangements with you to pay for the evaluation in increments.

> A *sliding scale* means that, based on your family income, the evaluator will adjust what she charges you for the evaluation.

Q: We've heard that one of the advantages of getting our child's evaluation done privately and not through the schools is that we control the results. Unless we give the report to the school, they never need to know about it. We don't understand why you wouldn't want the school to see the report, though–isn't the whole point to help her in school?

A: Yes, but there are circumstances in which families do not want to share all the content or even the results of certain evaluations. For example, a psychological testing report may include personal family history that they do not want to be part of the school's record on their child. Or the evaluation itself, such as a sexual abuse evaluation, may be considered too private to share with the school. Private evaluations also sometimes include a diagnosis, terms such as *attention-deficit/hyperactivity disorder* (ADHD), *Asperger syndrome*, or *obsessive–compulsive disorder* (OCD). Though we believe generally it is helpful to share this kind of information, some parents worry about "labeling" their children or are concerned about the stigma they think is attached to certain diagnoses.

Because we strongly believe that almost all types of evaluations have some important relevance to a child's functioning at school, we suggest that you ask the provider to edit out the sections that include personal information so that you will then feel comfortable sharing the report with the school. The edited information could include background, behavioral observations, or even diagnoses and recommendations (e.g., for psychotherapy or HIV testing). You can't ask the provider to change test scores, impressions, or conclusions, though.

It is important to note that any report you submit to the school *becomes a part of the child's permanent school record.* The school is obligated by law to keep such information confidential, however.

Q: What's the right way to give the school our son's evaluation report? Do we just bring it to his teacher?

A: You will usually want to have the teacher read the report, but you should also typically include the special education staff. If the results indicate any type of disability or weakness that might be suitable for an

IEP or a 504 Plan, you should contact the school's special education department and ask for a team meeting to review the report and discuss a plan. It is smart to give the school a copy of the report at least a week in advance so that the other team members have a chance to read it before the meeting. Depending on the flexibility of your school system, the team may or may not write up an IEP or Section 504 Plan at the meeting. As we mentioned before, some schools will insist on retesting your child to see for themselves what the problems may be. You should find out your school's policy on this *before* you have your child evaluated privately, so you can make a more informed choice about where to have him tested.

Q: *I know that the psychologist testing my daughter will meet with my husband and me after all the results are in. My daughter is ten years old, though, and I'm sure she'll be curious about how she did and what it all means for her. Does she meet with the psychologist, too?*

A: This really depends on the child, though it sounds as though your daughter will want some feedback. Often, the evaluator will give the child information as to how she is doing during the session, such as praise for a good job or good effort. At the end of the session, sometimes the evaluator may say something like, "I think we've figured out why reading is so tough for you and how to help." There will be times when it is appropriate for the child to be present at the parent feedback meeting or to meet with the evaluator separately. This is true for most kids in their teens and for children who seem especially nervous or curious about how they did and what happens next. We have had feedback meetings with kids that have been therapeutic because they were able to acknowledge their sadness or anger over a previously undiagnosed learning disability or feel relief that someone finally understood how hard things had been for them. The renewal of hope is also an important aspect of the feedback meeting for parents and kids. So, we generally recommend that children twelve and older, and even younger children when appropriate, meet, even briefly, with the evaluator to go over the evaluation.

Q: *In the recommendations section of my daughter's neuropsychological evaluation, the psychologist said that she should be tested again in about two years. Is that really necessary, or is the psychologist just trying to drum up business for herself?*

A: Though you are right to be a cautious consumer, it is not at all un-usual to recommend that a child receive follow-up testing in two to three years. Generally, the results of a neuropsychological evaluation are considered valid or current for up to three years. You do not have to use the same psychologist for the follow-up evaluation, but if you were pleased with the work she did this time, it is often a good idea to have the same provider for the follow-up. One reason is that your child will probably remember the office, if not the psychologist, which can increase his comfort level. Maybe more important, the psychologist will be familiar with your child, the school situation, and the com-munity supports he has been get-ting. She will also have the raw data from the previous evalua-tion available to her should she need to refer to it for any reason.

Raw data are the actual test response forms, notes, drawings, and any other in-formation obtained during the evaluation with your child. These are held as a confi-dential file by the evaluating psychologist for several years should you or the evalu-ator need them later.

Now You Know Where—But Who?

This chapter should have helped you decide which route to take—public or private—for your child's testing evaluation. As we've already pointed out, you do not get to choose the evaluator if you are having your child tested through public means (EI, the school system). However, it's a good idea to get a sense of all the possible players on your child's EI or school team; we cover this subject in the next chapter.

If you have decided to get a private evaluation, Chapter Three will also be of help to you in figuring out what all those different titles and letters mean—neurologist? psychologist? psychiatrist? MD? PhD? MSW? —as you look for the right professional with the right qualifications to work with your child.

Three

Who Is Qualified to Conduct the Evaluation?

Zach's mother, Tina, was finally convinced that pursuing testing for Zach was the right thing to do. Zach's behavior hadn't improved by the end of first grade, and his teacher was concerned about how he'd do in second grade. After his parents had explained Zach's difficulties in school to their pediatrician, the pediatrician suggested they get a private evaluation. The school was suggesting that the school psychologist do the evaluation. To confuse things even more, Tina's friends were providing her with the names and phone numbers of professionals they had used. Tina looked at the list of psychologists, neuropsychologists, psychiatrists, pediatric psychopharmacologists, social workers, and educational consultants. A year ago she hadn't known some of these professions even existed. Now she had to decide which one would be best to evaluate her child. When she called our office, her first question to our office staff was "Who is the best person to evaluate my son?"

Tina's question is not an easy one to answer, as the number of professionals available to test children can be quite overwhelming. We often hear questions such as, "What is the difference between a psychologist and a psychiatrist? A social worker and an educational consultant? A counselor and a school psychologist?" "How do I know the person I've chosen is the best available practitioner?" The most frequent question on this topic relates to a parent's ability to trust the person doing the testing and frequently sounds like, "How can I trust the tester? How do I know this person will do a good job and interpret the test results accurately?" Although we can't vouch for each and every evaluator, we can provide you with information that can help you make an informed and comfortable decision.

Clinical Psychologists

Today a variety of professionals offer help to people with psychological and learning problems; however, only a few of them are able to provide psychological testing. Most prominent in this group are *clinical psychologists*, professionals who earn a doctorate in clinical psychology by completing at least four to six years of graduate training in the diagnosis and treatment of psychological disorders, as well as a full-time, year-long internship at a hospital or mental health agency. As part of their education, most clinical psychologists receive training in statistics, research methods, and related subjects such as physiology and neurology. In addition, if they choose to specialize in certain topics (such as psychological assessment), they will have had practical experience at a school, hospital, or clinic, as well.

Not every clinical psychologist is competent at providing testing, because many clinical psychologists specialize instead in the treatment of psychological disorders. Other clinical psychologists are primarily researchers. Therefore, it is important for you to ask the person about his qualifications to provide testing. Your best guide in finding a competent psychologist may be to ask a professional that you already trust, such as your child's pediatrician or psychiatrist. If your child is already receiving counseling, it would be wise to ask your child's therapist for some names. Ask the referring doctor if she has ever worked with this psychologist and what the experience was like for the family and child.

Neuropsychologists

Neuropsychology is a subspecialty within psychology. Neuropsychologists are typically clinical psychologists who have received advanced postdoctoral training in neuropsychological testing. Although not medically trained, neuropsychologists do have training in neuroanatomy, physiology, and basic clinical neurology, in addition to more traditional clinical psychology. Because of this specialized training, the neuropsychologist's main area of interest and expertise is the relationship between behavior and abnormal brain function.

Neuropsychologists are not typically trained to do projective test-ing (or tests of psychological functioning), such as the Rorschach. If it has been recommended that your child receive tests of psychological or emotional functioning and you decide to see a neuropsychologist, you will want to ask whether he is qualified to give those tests. Sometimes neuropsychologists will collaborate with psychologists who are quali-fied to give projective tests. Other neuropsychologists have received training in both neuropsychological and psychological testing and will be qualified to do the entire evaluation.

If you were confined to choosing only one person to do an evalua-tion of your child's cognitive or academic functioning, you couldn't go wrong if you picked a competent neuropsychologist, as these practitio-ners' entire profession is dedicated to comprehensively evaluating chil-dren in the areas of cognition, academic achievement, memory, and neuropsychological functioning. If you are lucky enough to find a highly recommended neuropsychologist who is also trained to give pro-jective tests, you'll be able to feel confident that this person has the ability to evaluate your child's functioning in multiple areas.

Neuropsychologists are not typically employed in the schools, but some are well versed in school procedures and requirements. If you de-cide to have a private neuropsychologist evaluate your child, you should, in fact, ascertain whether the clinician is knowledgeable about working with schools. If you choose to have your child evaluated through the school system, on the other hand, the person most able to evaluate multiple areas of functioning will be the school psychologist.

School Psychologists

School psychologists perform tasks such as counseling students and ad-ministering tests, particularly tests of cognition and academic achieve-ment. School psychologists are important providers of testing, and many children who have academic problems will never need to see an-other professional for testing besides the school psychologist. If your child's school psychologist has tested your child and you are pleased with the type of help your child has received and the rate of progress your child is making, there is little need to see a clinical psychologist or neuropsychologist. However, most school psychologists do not diag-nose children. In other words, although they are quite qualified to as-sess children's progress, to determine areas of strength and weakness, and to make recommendations for remediation, they do not generally label problems (e.g., dyslexia, Asperger syndrome). If having a firm diagnosis is important to you, you may need to talk with an additional professional or to get an independent evaluation. If you are unclear about whether getting a firm diagnosis is important, see the sidebar.

When Is Getting a Firm Diagnosis Important?

- *When you want to make sure your child gets the best possible overall treatment.* The schools can provide accommodations and special education services for kids whose test results establish a need. But suppose it looks as though your child has ADHD. Extensive research has shown that kids with this disorder benefit most from a combination of medication and behavioral treatment (see Chapter Seven). Getting a firm diagnosis of ADHD will allow you to get a prescription for appropriate stimulant medications (many doctors will not prescribe medication without a firm diagnosis) and also behavioral therapy that you can use at home—both of which could make your child happier and healthier overall but also augment any improvements in school performance brought on by services the school is willing to deliver.
- *When you don't want to waste any time in getting help for your child.* Your child is more likely to get the assistance he needs *quickly* when a professional is able to determine exactly what's wrong. The American Psychiatric Association's *Diagnostic and Statistical Manual of Mental Disorders* (DSM-IV), now in its fourth edition, sharply defines the signs and symptoms of disorders through lists of criteria for diagnosis. Knowing that all of these symptoms may be affecting your child can help the professionals zero in on every intervention with the potential to help, from school accommodations to medication, psychological therapy, and social support. If your child has been suffering debilitating difficulties at home, at school, and with friends—and if you've already waited months for a testing evaluation to be completed—time may be of the essence.
- *When you want to be an active, informed participant in your child's treatment.* Without a firm diagnosis, you may have an idea of what's wrong with your child, but all you really have to work with is a collection of findings from the test results. You can research those findings individually, but if in fact the findings add up to a specific

diagnosis, having a name for your child's difficulties will make it easier for you to locate more information about your child's specific problems. Imagine how much time might be saved if you looked up "treatments for Asperger syndrome" rather than separately researching variously defined difficulties with assembling and building objects, interacting with others, and reading comprehension.

- *When the school seems to be on the fence about providing services for your child:* As we've said, no diagnosis is a guarantee that your child will receive assistance from the public schools, as that decision hinges on whether your child's school performance is suffering. But if test results are unclear, borderline, or otherwise questionable, receiving a firm diagnosis from an outside professional may just turn the decision in your child's favor. In addition, having a firm diagnosis may allow your child to get more appropriate services from the school system, eliminating the need for a certain amount of trial and error.

- *When you want your insurance plan to pay for various types of treatment for your child.* Many insurance plans mete out coverage for treatment such as private psychotherapy, speech and language therapy, and occupational therapy sparingly. In many cases, coverage will be denied altogether without a firm diagnosis as justification for the treatment.

Educational Psychologists

Educational psychologists are typically involved in improving curricula, teaching methods, and administration of academic programs. They are not typically trained to perform neuropsychological assessments. However, some of them may have received advanced training in assessment and, as a result, would be qualified to perform many of the tests mentioned in this book.

Educational psychologists and educational consultants, even those who do not perform testing, are sometimes involved in extended evaluations. For example, in our practice we may contract with an educational consultant to observe a child in a school or to represent our reports at an IEP meeting (see Chapter Two). At other times, we may make a referral to an educational consultant who can help parents decide which school will best meet their child's individual needs. The educational consultant uses the results of our evaluation, along with her knowledge about schools in the area, to help match the student with an appropriate educational environment.

Psychiatrists

The terms *psychiatrist* and *psychologist* are easy to confuse, as they often are used interchangeably in the vernacular. In reality, they are two quite different groups of professionals. Psychiatrists are physicians who, after completing medical school and receiving their MDs, go on to specialize in the treatment of mental disorders. Psychiatrists perform psychiatric evaluations with the purpose of providing a diagnosis for your child's difficulties. They may ask you detailed questions about your child's history and perform a physical examination and laboratory tests (particularly if they are planning on prescribing medication). *Psychopharmacology* is a subspecialty within psychiatry. Psychopharmacologists are psychiatrists who specialize in prescribing medication to treat psychiatric symptoms. Psychiatrists do not receive training in cognitive, academic, or neuropsychological testing. They can't tell you what your child's IQ is. They are, however, a potentially important part of your child's treatment team.

Q: Can I tell what type of doctor to see by the letters after the doctor's name?

A: Not necessarily. Although many evaluators will have PhDs, there are qualified individuals who have master's degrees. Much depends on the licensing requirement in the state in which the evaluator resides. For example, in some states one can be a licensed school psychologist with an MA. In other states a doctorate is needed. Your best bet is to find a licensed professional. See the sidebar "Questions to Ask Your Psychologist." Use the answers to determine whether you feel this person will work well with your child. Also see the sidebar "Making Sense of the Letters."

Questions to Ask Your Psychologist

- How many children have you seen who have problems like my son's or daughter's?
- How many years have you been in practice?
- Where did you receive your training in psychological testing?
- Do you have a subspecialty area? Do you have expertise in evaluating learning disabilities and developmental disorders?
- Do you have expertise in working with public school systems?
- In addition to diagnosing the problem, can you make specific recommendations regarding interventions and accommodations to me, as well as to teachers, school psychologists, and others who might be involved in helping my child?
- What type of degree do you have?
- Are you licensed?
- Do you typically evaluate children or adults?
- What types of tests are you planning to give to my child?
- Are you qualified to perform neuropsychological tests? Tests of emotional functioning?
- Are there types of evaluations you feel you are not qualified to perform?

Other Professionals

The following professionals do not perform neuropsychological or psychological evaluations. However, they have specialized skills in certain areas, and their focused evaluations are often included as part of a comprehensive evaluation. In addition, the results of a neuropsychological evaluation may indicate that further testing in one or more of these areas is indicated. As a result, your psychologist may recommend an additional evaluation by one or more of these professionals.

Speech and language pathologists perform a variety of roles for children who have speech and language disorders. In public schools, speech–language pathologists provide therapy (both within and outside the classroom) to children with communication disorders. They also evaluate speech and language difficulties in children, both as part of a school evaluation and within private settings.

Occupational therapists help individuals manage and remediate their difficulties. They may teach perceptual–motor, sensory integration, self-help, and daily living skills. They also evaluate these skills in children and adults.

Physical therapists provide services to restore or improve physical functioning, such as gross-motor coordination, range of motion, and movement. They are frequent evaluators of these skills in children.

School counselors are important resources in treating children with a variety of emotional and educational problems. They provide assistance when children have behavioral problems or crises and can be an

Making Sense of the Letters

PhD = Doctor of Philosophy
Includes clinical psychologists, school psychologists, counseling psychologists

MD = Doctor of Medicine
Includes psychiatrists and other medical doctors

PsyD = Doctor of Psychology
Includes some clinical psychologists who attended a graduate program with a curriculum that included less emphasis on teaching and research and more emphasis on therapeutic intervention

EdD = Doctorate in Education
Included in this group are some clinical psychologists and educational psychologists.

MA = Master of Arts

MS = Master of Science

MEd = Master of Education

MSW = Master of Social Work

LICSW = Licensed Clinical Social Worker

OTR = Registered Occupational Therapist

PT = Physical Therapist

CCC-SLP = Licensed Speech Therapist

Q: *I asked my child's pediatrician for the name of a neuropsychologist who could perform my child's evaluation. She highly recommended Dr. Sanderson. When I spoke to Dr. Sanderson, I really didn't get a good feel for him—we just didn't seem to connect. I also think my daughter would relate better to a female. Should I stick with the pediatrician's recommendation or trust my instinct and find someone else?*

A: If you're having doubts about a doctor you were referred to, you should probably get some other recommendations. It's important that you find someone with whom you feel comfortable. Although you want someone who is very skilled and knowledgeable, you also need to work well with this person and be able to relate to him on an emotional level. It's also important to consider whether your child would work better with a male or female evaluator. Most children can work well with either, but if they have a strong preference (sometimes as a result of a traumatic incident), it may make sense to honor their wishes.

Q: *My pediatrician recommended that Dr. Roome, a well-known neuropsychologist, evaluate my daughter. However, when I called Dr. Roome's office, her secretary told me that Dr. Roome's first appointment was five months away! She suggested that I see Dr. Roome's associate, who had an availability four weeks from now. Dr. Roome has such a great reputation—should I wait five months or take a chance with her associate?*

A: The answer to your question depends somewhat on how severe your child's difficulties are. Generally, parents who are seeking testing want it done as soon as possible. However, they also want to make sure that they see a reputable person. As a general rule, if Dr. Roome is well regarded, then likely others in her practice will be competent also. We would recommend speaking briefly with Dr. Roome's associate. Ask him about his training and qualifications. Describe your child's difficulties to him and ask him how he would approach the evaluation. Perhaps after speaking with him, you can get a better sense of whether this will be a good fit for your child.

Q: *When I called the neuropsychology department at my local hospital to make an appointment for my son, I was told that he would be evaluated by a psychology intern who is supervised by a licensed neuropsychologist. Is this ever a good idea?*

A: Yes, this is often a very good idea. Psychology interns are psychology students who have reached the end of their training and who are working in the field of psychology under close supervision. Sometimes a child receives a more thorough evaluation than if the child had been evaluated by a single neuropsychologist. For example, the interns will spend time in supervision with the supervising psychologist. They will thoroughly discuss your child's case and determine the types of tests that are needed, review the tests once they are completed, and determine diagnostic and treatment recommendations. Sometimes a child's case will be presented and discussed at a case conference, at which a team of professionals will review the test results.

When we supervise interns, we often have them perform *more* tests than we would complete if we were doing the testing, so that we get as complete a picture of the child as possible. We sometimes observe the intern complete the testing and often attend the feedback session. You should know that if you decide to have your child evaluated by a psychology trainee, you always have the option of talking with the intern's supervisor if you are unhappy with the evaluation or if you have questions that are answered insufficiently by the trainee.

Q: *My daughter needs to be tested for learning problems in school. We are a bilingual family and speak both Spanish and English. English is really a second language for my daughter, though she is fluent in it. Would there be any advantage in requesting a Spanish-speaking psychologist to do the evaluation? Will the psychologist be culturally sensitive when interpreting the results?*

A: This question comes up often when we work with bilingual children, especially if they are not yet fluent in English, the language they will be tested in unless otherwise arranged. Most large hospitals and clinics will have bilingual clinicians; if not, interpreter services can often be arranged with advance notice. If your child were not yet fluent in English, we would certainly recommend either finding a psychologist who speaks your child's primary language for the evaluation or having an interpreter assist the psychologist to make sure the results are as accurate as possible. Given that she speaks English as well as she does Spanish, there would not necessarily be any reason to have her tested in Spanish. This is particularly true if she attends an English-language school.

Whether or not the psychologist working with your child will be culturally sensitive when interpreting results is extremely variable, though now doctorate-level psychologists are required to take courses on ethnicity and cross-culturalism in graduate school. We strongly recommend that you discuss your concerns up front with the evaluator, making sure you emphasize how you feel your daughter's functioning in school may be affected by cultural differences (e.g., her answers are marked wrong when she occasionally exchanges a Spanish phrase for an English one; she feels left out when celebrating cultural holidays that are not also celebrated by her peers or talked about in school, etc.). If you feel that the clinician is not receptive to your input or seems to minimize your concerns, we advise you to choose another evaluator who will be more attuned to the importance of this issue.

---

important link among the classroom teacher, the principal, and parents. They are often involved in monitoring student progress and developing and implementing behavioral treatment plans.

As you may have guessed from reading this chapter, there is no one right person for every possible evaluation. If you'd like the evaluation to be completed through the school system, most likely a team of professionals—which could include a school psychologist, a speech and language therapist, an occupational therapist, a school guidance counselor, a reading specialist, and/or a physical therapist—will evaluate your child. If you decide to seek a private and comprehensive evaluation, you will probably want to begin with a neuropsychologist or clinical psychologist. However, the neuropsychologist will sometimes, depending on the difficulties seen in the evaluation, refer you for a more specialized evaluation from another professional, such as a speech and language or occupational therapist.

> Remember Zach from the beginning of this chapter? His mom knew pursuing an evaluation was the right thing to do but not how to find the right person to do it. After consulting with Zach's pediatrician and school personnel, she decided to engage the services of a private neuropsychologist who was highly recommended. She also decided to have Zach's fine-motor and language skills testing completed by the school's occupational therapist and speech and language therapist. Additionally, she met with the school psychologist and guidance counselor during the team meeting held to review the results.
>
> Tina felt confident that she had made the right decision. She liked the fact that the neuropsychologist could give her a firm diagnosis of Zach's disability. Because the neuropsychologist diagnosed Zach

with ADHD, Tina could take the neuropsychologist's report to Zach's pediatrician, who then could discuss the pros and cons of medication with Tina and her husband, David. Tina also liked the fact that the school evaluated some areas of Zach's functioning. As it turned out, Zach's fine-motor skills were weak, and he could benefit from occupational therapy. The occupational therapist who evaluated Zach began treating him soon after completing the evaluation and was already familiar with his skill weaknesses. Zach was comfortable with her and was easily engaged in the treatment process.

Tina's friend, Helen, made a different decision for her son, Jason. Jason's difficulties were in the area of reading. School personnel evaluated Jason when he was in the second grade, and their assessment indicated that he needed intensive tutoring in reading. The school provided this tutoring four times a week and gave Jason additional academic resource-room support. Helen was satisfied with the evaluation and the progress Jason was making and never decided to pursue additional testing.

Diane pursued a totally different course of action for her daughter Sarah, who was struggling to keep up with grade-level reading assignments in the third grade at an elite private school. Diane took Sarah to a neuropsychologist, who diagnosed Sarah with mild dyslexia. Although Diane was happy to have a firm diagnosis, she did not want the school to see a copy of the report, because she was afraid the school might ask Sarah to leave. Instead, she decided to pay for intensive private tutoring and asked the neuropsychologist to write a letter to the school indicating some strategies that might be helpful for Sarah in the classroom. Because Sarah's dyslexia was mild, she was able to cope with the demands of school, and she made good progress.

Although these families chose different evaluations for their children and were pleased with the eventual outcome, they all had one common experience. Each of them was given a report, or reports, that explained their children's functioning. Unfortunately, these reports, which they had hoped would answer all their questions about their children's problems, only raised additional questions. What were all the tests mentioned in the report? What had they measured? How could the parents interpret the confusing array of scores and percentages included in the report? The next two chapters help answer these questions.

Part II

A Practical Guide to Commonly Used Tests

Four

The Tests: What Are They and What Do They Do?

Zach and his mother arrived early for his appointment, and it was easy to see that Zach was nervous, maybe even a little scared. His mother explained, "I didn't know what to tell him about what he'd be doing today. I wish I had asked more questions about what the tests would involve, because when I couldn't explain exactly what he'd be asked to do, Zach got angry and didn't want to come. Can you tell us more about the tests before we start—and help Zach understand what it will be like for him?"

This scenario is so typical that we always schedule some time before administering the tests for a kind of orientation, for both the child and the parents. In many cases, parents who have gone through the often protracted process of arranging for a testing evaluation—from making the initial decision to have a child tested to choosing between school and private testing to locating the best evaluators and getting an appointment—end up making the appointment for the child without ever having spoken with the psychologist who will be performing the testing. Sometimes they're motivated by simple trust in the experts and sometimes they have a mental image of what testing will involve and feel no need to elaborate on it. We strongly encourage you to speak to the evaluator at some point before your child's evaluation, if for no other reason than to break the ice, but especially because kids often surprise Mom and Dad with last-minute questions, and they'll be much more relaxed about this noninvasive assessment if you can tell them accurately what to expect. Ask what tests the evaluator plans to do and why. Find out what your child will be asked to do, how long the tests should take, and whether there is anything you should do to prepare your child (or yourself). We include some suggestions for preparing for testing in each chapter of Part III.

The purpose of this chapter is to explain some of the most common tests used in psychological, educational, and neuropsychological evaluations. Reading this chapter won't make you an expert on testing. It can, however, help you prepare your child for the test session and also help you understand the results after the test process is completed. Once you know what tests the evaluator has scheduled for your child, look up the tests in this chapter so that you'll have a better idea of what to expect at the appointment. If your child has already been evaluated, you can use this chapter as a handy reference for understanding particular tests long after the evaluation is completed. If you're in the process of deciding whether your child needs an evaluation, use this chapter to learn more about what the tests actually do—this may help guide your decision as to whether testing is the answer to your child's difficulties.

In addition to the tests described in this chapter, you'll find more information about tests used to evaluate specific disorders in Part III of this book. So, for example, if you're concerned that your child may have dyslexia, read Chapter Six for a description of the specific tests that are used to diagnose dyslexia.

In general, tests are used to gather information about certain aspects of a person's functioning. This information is often used to make broader interpretations about that person's ability to function in other areas of life. For Zach, a hyperactive, inattentive first-grader, testing can be used to determine whether he has the cognitive ability and academic skills to be successful in first grade. It can determine whether his difficulties are due to problems with focused attention or to an underlying learning disability. The evaluation can assess whether his hyperactivity is typical for boys his age or whether it is out of the range of normal and worthy of treatment.

The tests that clinicians use to diagnose these and other problem behaviors typically fall into one of the following categories, in the order in which an evaluation is often completed. For example, a clinical interview is often the first step in the diagnostic process because it provides general information about a child's history and reason for referral. Intelligence and achievement tests are almost always part of a comprehensive evaluation. The last three categories include tests that an evaluator may or may not elect to use.

1. *Clinical interviews* typically involve asking the child or parent a series of questions. Clinical interviews can range from very informal to very structured.
2. *Intelligence tests* are used to measure a person's intellectual ability, such as the ability to apply information in new and different ways.
3. *Achievement tests* are used to measure a person's achievement in subjects such as math, reading, and writing, including spelling, punctuation, writing expression, and so forth.
4. *Neuropsychological tests* assess brain functioning in areas such as language, auditory perception, verbal and visual memory, and perceptual–motor speed and integration.
5. *Projective tests and tests of emotional functioning* are used to assess psychological functioning.
6. *Self-report and behavioral rating measures* consist of lists of items, or checklists, that people are asked to endorse as either true or false, for themselves or for the person being observed.

Depending on the particular concerns about the child, the evaluator may use some or all of these measures. The choice of tests and the order in which they are administered are decisions that need to be made on an individual basis, taking into consideration your concerns, the age

> *Neuropsychological tests* differ from a *neuropsychological evaluation.* Neuropsychological tests are specific types of tests, whereas a neuropsychological evaluation will include tests from categories 1 through 4, as well as (sometimes) measures from categories 5 and 6.

of your child, previous test results, whether your child is also being evaluated in the schools, and so forth. For example, if your second-grade child is struggling with reading but is having no other difficulties in school or in social relationships, the examiner may choose to administer an IQ test, tests of achievement (with a particular emphasis on reading measures), and a measure or two of behavioral functioning. However, another second-grade child who is having difficulty reading may also be having trouble concentrating and may be exhibiting signs of depression. In that case, the examiner may, in addition to the tests just mentioned, choose to administer some neuropsychological measures (to assess attention, concentration, and memory), as well as some projective tests. Because there is no "one size fits all" test battery, it is important to make sure that you have chosen a competent examiner who will administer the tests that will address your concerns (see Chapter Two for more information about this). If, at the end of the evaluation process, your questions have been answered and appropriate treatment recommendations have been made, you can feel confident that the examiner competently completed the evaluation.

Clinical Interviews

The clinical interview is often the first contact between the parent and child and the clinician. The purpose of the clinical interview is to obtain detailed information about the person's current problems and feelings, developmental and medical histories, school and academic histories, family and social relationship histories, and current level of functioning. Interviews can be either structured or unstructured. In unstructured interviews the clinician asks open-ended questions, such as, "Tell me what prompted you to bring Bobby in for an evaluation." In a structured interview the clinician asks a standard set of questions or addresses topics that are used for everyone. Structured interviews sometimes include a mental status exam, interview questions, and observations designed to determine a person's precise level of functioning. The questions generally cover areas of functioning such as an awareness of one's surroundings, orientation to time and place, attention span, auditory memory, thought content and mood, and appearance.

Most clinicians will use a combination of structured and unstructured formats. It is common for a psychologist or clinic to ask you to complete a formal intake evaluation that will include structured questions. Many clinicians will follow this up with a less structured face-to-face interview with the parent and child. Typically the clinician will want to speak to the parent and child separately.

Structured interviews include a standard set of questions that are administered orally to individuals.

The interview is very important because it frames the evaluation process. That is, it provides clinicians with information that allows them to make hypotheses about what may be underlying a child's difficulties. These hypotheses are used to determine what tests may be most useful and what areas of functioning should be examined most closely. For example, Zach's mother indicated during the clinical interview and on the structured intake form that Zach was a "difficult baby who grew up to be a rambunctious toddler." She noted in his developmental history that he was extremely active and had difficulty paying attention and gave many examples of how these behaviors have become a problem for him. She indicated that Zach had few difficulties learning the content of academic subjects but said, "He just can never sit still long enough to complete an assignment." After listening to her detailed history, the clinician knew that she needed to thoroughly evaluate Zach's attention and organizational skills.

Intelligence Tests

Probably no other single area of testing has seen more controversy than that of intelligence. Psychologists have debated whether intelligence is learned or inherited, culturally specific or universal, one ability or several abilities. These debates are ongoing and won't soon be resolved. For our purposes, however, we discuss intelligence as it relates to a child's score on an IQ test. Efforts to measure intelligence have long been a part of psychology. Although still surrounded by controversy, IQ tests are the most studied, and consequently the most reliable, valid, and useful, tests available. Within a test, people tend to perform the same on items designed to assess the same ability, thus suggesting internal consistency. They are reliable because people will generally get the same score when they retake the same test years later. Studies that have compared children's IQ scores with their performance in school have found that IQ and school performance are highly correlated. That is, they are one of the best single indices of how well a child will do in school. Having said that, IQ tests are not the sole factor determining how a person will perform in school and are not the definitive indication of how a person will eventually function in society, as other variables, such as parenting, quality of schooling, motivation, and exposure to culture and books, are also important determinants of success in life.

An IQ score reflects a person's performance on an intelligence test relative to that of persons the same age. We'll explain more about how this is done in Chapter Five, but, in short, a child's IQ score tells you the extent to which his performance on the test departs from average.

Nearly all comprehensive evaluations include some measure of intelligence. For example, for a child who is being tested to confirm a diagnosis of ADHD, an intelligence test can determine that the child's academic difficulties don't come from a specific cognitive weakness or mild mental retardation. An intelligence test is absolutely necessary to diagnose any type of learning disability because by definition a learning disability is a noteworthy discrepancy between a child's cognitive ability (i.e., intelligence) and academic achievement.

Despite their limitations, IQ tests are the best measure we have of a person's abilities in a variety of areas. Because they test multiple areas, IQ tests are composed of subtests that measure more specific abilities. Scores on these subtests are combined to yield measures of verbal and performance abilities, as well as a Full Scale IQ score.

The most common intelligence tests for children include the following:

WPPSI-III, WISC-III, and WAIS-III IQ Scores

Verbal IQ includes items that assess abilities such as vocabulary, arithmetic skills, short-term memory performance, and knowledge of general information.

Performance IQ includes tests of visual–spatial skills, puzzle assembly, and nonverbal reasoning.

Full Scale IQ is a composite of the two scales. In addition to providing the information for which the tests were designed, the Full Scale IQ also opens a window into a variety of cognitive functions, such as memory and sequencing.

Wechsler Intelligence Scale for Children—Third Edition (WISC-III) and Fourth Edition (WISC-IV)

The Wechsler Intelligence Scale for Children is the most widely used test of intelligence for children ages six through sixteen years. There are currently two different editions of the WISC. The WISC-IV is the newest version of the WISC available in the fall of 2003, at which time the use of the WISC-III will fade out. It can take a year or two from publication of a new version of the WISC for professionals to become trained on the newer version. Thus, we provide information about both versions of the test, as we're expecting that both versions will be used for a year or so after this book is published. However, don't expect to see the WISC-III in use much after 2004.

WISC-IV

The WISC-IV includes numerous subtests and yields only a Full Scale IQ score. The WISC-IV also yields four "factor scores," which measure different dimensions of functioning. These factor scores are Verbal Comprehension, Perceptual Reasoning, Processing Speed, and Working Memory. They and are derived from select verbal and nonverbal subtests. These factors reflect a child's performance on meaningful dimensions of mental ability and provide useful information regarding a child's learning style. The Verbal Comprehension factor measures children's verbal knowledge and their ability to use their verbal skills in new situations. Scores on this factor are also a reflection of a child's educational and home environments. In other words, if a child is surrounded by an environment that is verbally enriched, he will likely do well or better on this factor. The Perceptual Reasoning factor reflects the ability to think about and organize visual material without the use of words. Processing Speed measures the speed at which children can process simple visual information, such as abstract design or numbers, without making errors. Although it is not a measure of a child's ability to think or reason, difficulty in processing simple information (e.g., copying symbols or letters or quickly scanning a work sheet for mistakes) leaves a child with less time and mental energy to understand and process new material. Working Memory is an indication of a child's ability to hold information in memory so that he can manipulate it or perform calculations with it. It includes the ability to do mental arithmetic and is affected by poor attention.

Verbal Subtests

The verbal subtests include:

> *Vocabulary,* a test in which the child is asked to define words of increasing difficulty (e.g., "What is a cat?" or "What does *frustrated* mean?"). This is a test of word knowledge, learning ability, and language development.

> *Information,* in which the child is asked to answer a wide range of questions that tap general knowledge, such as "Who was Mozart?" The test is designed to sample the knowledge that average children with average opportunities should be able to acquire. However, this test is influenced by opportunities both inside and outside the home, and low scores are not necessarily an indication of innate ability.

> *Similarities,* in which the child is asked how two things go together, such as "In what way are a dress and pants the same?" This is a test of verbal concept formation, or the ability to meaningfully place things or objects together in groups.

Arithmetic, in which the child is asked to solve simple arithmetic problems that have been read by the examiner (e.g., "If eggs cost $1.20 a dozen, how much does one egg cost?"). This

> **Working memory** is the ability to remember something while you're working on something else, such as the ability to do mental math. It functions very much like the brain's "scratch pad."

is an oral test in which the child does not have the advantage of using paper and pencil to help with solving the problems. As such, it is not only a measure of math ability but also an important measure of attention and concentration.

Comprehension, in which the child is asked to provide answers to common social dilemmas or problems, such as "Why would a person buy flood insurance?" or "Why do we wear hats when it's cold outside?" This is a measure of a child's verbally expressed knowledge of conventional standards of behavior, social judgment, and common sense.

Digit Span, a test in which the child is asked to recall a series of numbers read by the examiner forward and backward. This is a test of short-term auditory memory and attention and mental control and manipulation.

Word Reasoning, a measure of verbal reasoning ability in which a child identifies an underlying concept given successive clues.

Letter–Number Sequencing, a measure of working memory in which the child hears a string of mixed-up numbers and letters and then has to repeat the numbers first in numerical order followed by the letters in alphabetical order.

Nonverbal Subtests

The nonverbal subtests include:

Block Design, in which red and white designs are shown on cards and the child is asked to reproduce the designs using blocks. It is a measure of spatial visualization, perceptual organization, and abstract conceptualization. It also measures motor speed, as it is a timed test.

Picture Completion, a test of a child's ability to attend to visual details. Here, the child is shown colorful pictures and must identify the important missing detail in each.

Coding, a test of a child's ability to learn an unfamiliar task. On this test the child is asked to copy symbols paired with other symbols. The subtest is a measure of speed and accuracy of visual–motor coordination, attention, and short-term visual memory.

Symbol Search, a test of visual discrimination and visual–perceptual scanning ability in which the child is asked to look at a target symbol, as well as a group of symbols, and must decide quickly whether the target symbol is included in the group of symbols.

Matrix Reasoning, a measure of nonverbal reasoning in which the child is presented with an incomplete design or grid and is then asked to find the piece (from a group) that correctly completes the matrix.

Picture Concepts, a measure of perceptual organization, nonverbal reasoning, and the ability to categorize objects in which the child is asked to select objects that go together based on an underlying concept.

Cancellation, a measure of processing speed in which the child has to cross out certain objects on a page.

WISC-III

The WISC-III contains a few subtests that have been eliminated on the WISC-IV. They are:

Mazes, a test in which the child is asked to solve mazes that become increasingly complex. It is a measure of motor planning ability, as well as a measure of the ability to follow a visual pattern.

Picture Arrangement, in which the child is asked to arrange picture cards to tell a story that makes sense. It is a measure of visual discrimination and sequencing and requires concentration and quick motor speed, as it is a timed test. It is sometimes used to evaluate a child's nonverbal understanding of cause and effect in social situations.

Q: *My daughter's scores on the WISC-III indicated that she had a "15-point Verbal–Performance split." What does this mean, and should I be worried?*

A: In general, we expect children's verbal and performance abilities to be very similar. When differences are greater than 12 points, we consider that difference worthy of an explanation, but not necessarily cause for concern. Many learning disabilities result in large verbal–nonverbal splits on IQ tests. For example, many children with dyslexia will have lower verbal abilities because dyslexia is a verbally based learning disability. Children with nonverbal learning disabilities, by definition, have lower nonverbal IQ scores. However, a 15-point difference does not necessarily indicate the presence of a learning disability. Differences in styles of thinking and learning are extremely common and often reflected in a child's pattern of IQ scores. If an extremely large (over 25-point) verbal–nonverbal split exists, we often refer a child to a neurologist to rule out the possibility of neurological impairment. Even if there is a large difference, the discrepancy should not be used alone to make diagnoses or predictions about brain functioning without substantial support from other test data and observations.

Wechsler Adult Intelligence Scale—Third Edition (WAIS-III)

The WAIS-III is the most commonly used test of intelligence for persons ages sixteen through seventy-four years and may be the intelligence test chosen if your child is a teenager. The subtests on the WAIS-III are "adult" versions of the subtests on the WISC-IV.

Wechsler Preschool and Primary Scale of Intelligence—Third Edition (WPPSI-III)

This test is one of the most widely used tests of cognitive ability for young children, ages two and a half years to seven years, three months. It includes subtests that are similar in nature to those of the WISC-IV and WAIS-III and includes a Verbal and a Performance scale. Essentially, the WPPSI-III can be considered a downward extension of the WISC-IV. Because there is so much overlap between the

WPPSI-III and the WISC-IV, much of the information on the WISC-IV applies to the WPPSI-III. However, there are a couple of subtests that are unique to the WPPSI-III and that measure skills typically acquired during the preschool years. The subtests unique to the WPPSI-III are:

> *Receptive Vocabulary*, in which the child looks at a group of four pictures and points to the one named by the examiner. It is a measure of receptive language ability.

> *Picture Naming*, in which the child names a picture that is shown to him. It is a test of expressive language ability.

Wechsler Abbreviated Scale of Intelligence (WASI)

The WASI is a short measure of intelligence that can be used with individuals ages six to eighty-nine years. It yields Verbal, Performance, and Full Scale IQ scores. The WASI consists of four subtests: Vocabulary, Block Design, Similarities, and Matrix Reasoning. These subtests are similar to those described previously and were chosen because they have the highest correlation with general cognitive abilities. This test is often used when time is of concern, such as when insurance has restricted the number of billable hours or when children have health problems that may make a full IQ test too taxing for them. This test has limitations, of course; it is not going to be able to discern precise cognitive functioning and processing deficits and therefore may be less useful in diagnosing learning disabilities and other disorders.

Stanford–Binet Intelligence Scales, Fourth Edition

The Stanford–Binet IV can be used with individuals ages two through adulthood. It includes a battery of fifteen subtests, many of which are similar in content to those on the Wechsler scales. It measures four content areas: verbal reasoning (the ability to comprehend and use language appropriately), abstract/visual reasoning (the ability to reason without the use of words), quantitative reasoning (the ability to solve quantitative problems), and short-term memory (the ability to remember visual and verbal stimuli, such as a string of numbers or a visual picture). A general composite score is also obtained as a measure of overall intelligence.

Differential Ability Scales (DAS)

The DAS is a relatively recent test of cognitive ability for children ages two years, six months, through seventeen years, eleven months. It was devised to measure specific abilities across a range of cognitive domains, such as inductive reasoning ability, verbal ability, and spatial ability. It is similar to the Wechsler scales in a number of ways (e.g., it includes numerous subtests) but differs from it in other ways (e.g., the cognitive and achievement measures of the DAS were developed and normed together so that ability–achievement differences can be interpreted directly). The DAS yields a general conceptual ability score (GCA), which is similar but not identical to the Full Scale IQ of the WISC. The DAS also yields a verbal ability score, as well as two measures of nonverbal ability: nonverbal reasoning and spatial ability (the ability to perceive and remember spatial relationships and shapes, as well as analytical thinking and attention to visual detail).

Kaufman Assessment Battery for Children (K-ABC)

The K-ABC measures intelligence in children from ages two and a half through twelve years. It includes four scales that are a composite of different subtests: a sequential processing scale (measures a child's ability to solve problems that require arranging things in sequential or serial order); a simultaneous processing scale (measures a child's ability to solve problems that require the processing of many things at the same time, such as selecting a photograph of a face previously seen from a group of photographs or reproducing a design by using plastic triangles); an achievement scale (measures a child's factual knowledge and skills in things such as vocabulary use and understanding, reading, and arithmetic), and a nonverbal scale (composed of subtests that do not require words and thus are a measure of a child's nonverbal problem-solving ability). Although the K-ABC is useful in certain settings (particularly when information is needed about a child's nonverbal cognitive abilities), it is not generally used as the primary measure of a child's intellectual ability in clinical assessments.

Bayley Scales of Infant Development, Second Edition

The Bayley Scales of Infant Development is a commonly used measure of infant development for children from ages two months to three and a half years. It consists of three scales: a mental scale, a motor scale, and a behavior rating scale. The mental scale includes items such as looking for a fallen object, uncovering a toy, building a tower with blocks, imitating a crayon stroke, and naming pictures. The motor scale assesses fine-motor skills such as grasping or writing, as well as gross-motor skills such as sitting, walking, and jumping. Although the Bayley is an excellent measure of infant development, it is not a good predictor of intelligence, at least for samples of normal babies. The reason for this is thought to be that infant perceptual and motor behaviors don't represent the same aspects of intelligence that we assess on IQ tests in childhood. Tests of infant development are best used as screening instruments, helping to identify infants who need further observation and/or intervention because they may be more likely than others to experience future developmental problems.

Q: *With all of these measures of intelligence, how do I know the examiner gave my child the one that was best for her? My daughter scored in the average range on the WISC. Would she have done better on a different test? Should I have requested a particular test?*

A: There are indeed a number of good measures of cognitive ability, and each has pluses and minuses. However, the tests have more similarities than differences, and most children will get similar scores across the tests. The major exception to this rule would be a case in which an examiner gave a child an outdated version of the test. In this case, your child will likely do better on an outdated version, for complex reasons that are beyond the scope of this book. However, before you request your child be tested using an outdated version, you should be aware that no licensed professional should ethically do that, nor would most schools accept those results.

The examiner should have put much thought into picking the correct tests for your child, much as a physician picks the correct medicine to treat certain symptoms. It's usually not a good idea to ask for a certain test, unless you know that the child's school will accept results of only certain tests. For example, your local school district may require all children to be evaluated using the WISC-IV. In this case, it's essential that you inform the examiner of any specific required tests before the scheduled assessment.

Q: *Are any of the IQ tests you've listed favored by schools or private evaluators?*

A: There's no exact answer to this question, as there are no statistics on this. However, it's been our experience that schools—and private evaluators—most often use one of the Wechsler intelligence measures.

Q: *Is it advisable for my child to have more than one IQ test during the same evaluation process?*

A: It is rarely, if ever, advisable for a child to have more than one IQ test completed within a short period of time. IQ tests are quite stable—you generally see very similar scores across test situations and evaluators. The only reason to have more than one IQ test administered would be your belief that the testing is invalid. Invalid test results can occur if the evaluator is poorly trained or if the circumstances aren't conducive to test taking, such as the child being quite sick on the day of testing. If you have reason to believe the test results are invalid, talk with the examiner about your concerns and the pros and cons of getting a second test completed. Nearly always, the examiner would use a different IQ test, as giving the child the same IQ test in a short period of time would result in a questionably valid score.

Q: *My four-year-old, Linea, had an IQ test as part of an early intervention evaluation. She did worse on this test than we expected. How likely is it that her IQ will always be in this range?*

A: It's difficult to predict at age four what Linea's exact IQ will be at age fourteen. IQs are generally quite stable, but there are exceptions to every rule. The general rule of thumb is that the older the child, the more stable the IQ score. Tests such as the Bayley are not strongly related to later IQs, but correlations between adjacent-year IQ scores in middle childhood are quite high. However, although most older children show little fluctuation in their IQ scores, research has indicated that there is a subset of children who show wide fluctuation in their IQ scores. These wide fluctuations are more common in younger children.

In addition, older children may show some fluctuation in scores in response to major stressors such as loss of a parent, divorce, or a change in schools. With these possible exceptions, by age ten or so, IQ scores are highly stable. Our advice to you would be to continue to foster Linea's development and to provide her with opportunities for learning.

Achievement Tests

Achievement tests are designed to measure what a child has actually learned, including how well a child adds or subtracts, reads, spells, or understands science concepts. Most achievement tests focus on a particular subject and measure children's learning with questions of varying difficulty. The child's score is then either compared with that of a child the same age or grade or measured against some objective standard. For instance, the spelling achievement of Zach, a seven-year-old first grader, might be compared with that of other first graders or other seven-year-olds (some of whom may be in second grade) or with some general standard (such as a list of one hundred words that children in his particular state or school district are expected to know). Ideally, achievement tests should reveal not only what Zach has learned but also his weaknesses in specific skills or subject areas. For example, a math test might show that he has good computational skills but a poor understanding of time.

Achievement tests can sometimes be used to determine grade placement or to group students according to achievement level within each grade. These tests are also used by administrators or governmental agencies to evaluate the performance of teachers, schools, or school systems. Whether these are appropriate uses of achievement measures is debatable, because a child's performance on these tests can be affected by factors other than actual learning. When a psychologist administers an achievement test as part of a test battery, she is most interested in determining a person's areas of strengths and weaknesses, evaluating whether a learning disability exists, and determining whether a child is receiving adequate, appropriate instruction.

The more commonly used achievement tests include the following:

Wechsler Individual Achievement Test—Second Edition (WIAT-II)

The WIAT-II is an individually administered test for assessing the achievement of those ages four through adulthood. It measures content in the domains of reading, writing, mathematics, and oral language.

Wide Range Achievement Test 3 (WRAT3)

The WRAT3 consists of three subtests: reading, spelling, and arithmetic. The reading subtest asks the child to recognize and name letters and pronounce words. The spelling subtest measures the ability to copy letters, write one's name, and correctly spell dictated words. The arithmetic subtest measures skills such as reading numbers and solving written math problems, using addition, subtraction, multiplication, and division.

Woodcock–Johnson Psycho-Educational Battery—Revised or Third Edition (WJ-R) or (WJ-III)

This is a commonly used test of achievement, particularly in schools. It is a comprehensive battery that is administered individually. The battery can be administered to individuals from ages three years through adulthood and evaluates academic achievement in reading (including single-word reading, reading comprehension, and nonword reading), spelling, writing, and knowledge of science, humanities, social studies, and math.

Neuropsychological Tests

Neuropsychological tests are measures of sensorimotor, perceptual, language, and memory skills. A full listing of neuropsychological measures would fill this book, as literally hundreds of tests are available. Many clinicians use a battery of neuropsychological tests, each of which targets a specific cognitive skill area, such as memory, attention, and so forth. Research has shown that tests such as these can be valid in the assessment of brain damage and helpful in locating the area of the brain that has been affected. Performance on the tests is interpreted in light of what is known about the relation between certain brain structures and behaviors. For example, our abilities to tap a finger quickly, to speak, or to remember something are controlled by different areas of the brain. Thus the pattern of scores on various tests can tell us whether certain areas of the brain are impaired. This can be useful

Sensorimotor skills are the abilities involved in coordinating sensations with physical movements and actions.

Perceptual skills are the processes by which we organize and interpret sensory information.

in cases of brain injury, such as head trauma or brain tumors, when a doctor wants to identify which area of the brain is affected. However, neuropsychological tests are also used to further explore children's areas of strength and weakness—even in the absence of a traumatic injury. In other words, neuropsychological tests can determine whether a child has significant difficulties in areas such as language processing, attention, or visual–motor skills. These tests are commonly used when diagnosing learning disabilities and developmental delays.

The amount of time it takes to complete neuropsychological tests varies considerably. Most neuropsychological tests are brief measures of specific areas of functioning. Some tests can be completed in a matter of minutes, and others can take a half hour or more. The total length of testing depends on the number of tests given and the age of the child. Generally, the younger the child, the shorter the test period. If your child is scheduled for a "full neuropsychological evaluation," the evaluator will likely spend about one to two and a half hours completing these measures. (This time is in addition to the one to two hours spent administering an IQ test and one to two hours spent administering the achievement measures.) This is not the total of billable hours, as billable hours also include report writing, interpretation, scoring, consulting with teachers, and so forth. Thus the entire process generally takes from ten to sixteen hours. As a result, neuropsychological testing is often both extensive and expensive. As we've indicated before, a complete neuropsychological evaluation typically costs $1,500 to $2,500 or more, depending on the area of the country.

The tests that a neuropsychologist will choose to use depend in large part on the referral question. For example, if a child is reporting memory problems (perhaps as a result of an injury sustained in a car accident), the psychologist will likely focus on this area of functioning by giving the child a battery of memory tests that assesses the child's ability to recall information given to the child verbally (such as a string of numbers or a short story) or to recall something she's seen (such as a face or a design). If the referral question relates to attentional issues, the psychologist will likely give tests that will assess this area in particular. For example, tests of attention would include measures of a child's ability to listen to and recall a story, to attend to a computer stimulus, or to sustain attention through a repetitive task. Most neuropsychologists will pick and choose various neuropsychological tests, depending on the child and the referral question. However, there are also some standard batteries (collections of tests) that can be given.

One of the newest neuropsychological test batteries for children is the NEPSY. *NEPSY* is an acronym that was formed from the words *neuropsychology* and *psychology* (*NE-PSY*). The subtests of the NEPSY were designed for children between the ages of three and twelve. The subtests assess neuropsychological development in five areas: attention/executive functions, language, sensorimotor functions, visuospatial processing, and memory and learning. The battery was designed to assess cognitive abilities that are important to children's capacity to learn and be productive both in and out of school.

There is a fair amount of overlap between the skills measured on the NEPSY and a standard IQ test. However, IQ tests are designed primarily as measures of knowledge, reasoning, and judgment that yield a global measure of a child's functioning, whereas neuropsychological tests are designed to measure specific areas of functioning. Neuropsychological tests won't provide you with one number that summarizes a child's functioning in a number of different areas, as an IQ test does. Instead, each test measures a very small aspect of functioning (such as a person's ability to reproduce a drawing, put pegs in a hole, or remember a sentence), and it is the constellation of test results that is meaningful.

As mentioned earlier, many neuropsychologists won't give a standard battery but will pick and choose tests depending on the area they are most interested in assessing. Their choices of tests depend on an almost unlimited list of variables that includes things such as the referral question; whether the child has had previous testing and, if so, what the results indicated; when the previous testing was completed (if recently, they may choose not to repeat some measures); the age of the child; and the child's grade placement. Following are some of the more commonly used tests of neuropsychological, language, and memory functions. You can find out more about how and when these tests are used to diagnose particular disorders in Part III of this book. For now, we briefly present some of the more commonly used tests. Although the tests are categorized, most of them tap more than one specific area.

Language Tests

The *Boston Naming Test (BNT)* is a test of expressive vocabulary in which the child is presented with a series of line drawings of objects and, for each one, is asked to provide its name (e.g., *trumpet, elephant, broccoli*).

On the *Expressive One-Word Picture Vocabulary Test, Revised* (EOWPVT-R), the child is asked to name a series of pictured objects. It is a measure of single-word expressive vocabulary.

On the *Expressive Vocabulary Test* (EVT), the child is shown a series of pictures, one at a time. For each picture, a word is provided to describe the picture, and the child is asked to give another word that means the same thing as the word provided.

The *Clinical Evaluation of Language Functioning* (CELF-3) is a test that evaluates language skills in children and young adults, ages six through twenty-one years. It contains eleven subtests that evaluate various areas of language, such as auditory memory and expressive and receptive language skills. This test is rarely given in its entirety during a neuropsychological evaluation. Instead, the psychologist will use certain subtests as supplemental measures of language. In contrast, it is frequently given in its entirety during speech and language evaluations.

> *Expressive language* is the ability to use spoken language. *Receptive language* is the ability to comprehend or understand spoken language.

The *Peabody Picture Vocabulary Test* (PPVT-III) is a measure of single-word comprehension in which the child is read a series of words aloud and, for each one, is asked to determine which of four pictures portrays its meaning.

Tests of Memory

A number of batteries assess memory functioning, such as the *Children's Memory Scale (CMS)* and the *Wide Range Assessment of Memory and Learning* (WRAML). These test batteries include measures of memory in visual and verbal modalities and in immediate- and delayed-recall conditions. Memory is important to nearly all aspects of learning, so it is often assessed in an evaluation. However, sometimes memory problems are the primary focus of the testing, as in the case of memory loss as the result of a traumatic brain injury. Individuals experiencing a severe depression will also often report significant memory loss, and it is important to determine whether the memory difficulties are a result of the depression or have an organic cause (e.g., brain tumor). The subtests included in the verbal memory scale of the CMS include a measure of story memory, in which the child listens to two short stories and, immediately after hearing them and again after a delay, the child is asked to recall the story. On the word-pair subtest, word pairs are presented over three repeated trials; memory is tested after each of the trials by cueing with the first word in each pair and by free-recall condition in immediate- and delayed-recall conditions. Examiners will often administer parts of these batteries, depending on the areas they are most interested in examining.

The *Children's Auditory Verbal Learning Test (CAVLT)* and the *California Test of Verbal Learning–Children's Version (CVLT-C)* are tests of learning and memory. On this test, the child is asked to recall a list of fifteen or sixteen items presented repeatedly over five learning trials. Memory for the list is tested after each presentation; following the presentation of a different interference list (i.e., short delay); and again after a long delay, such as of thirty minutes or so, in free-recall (e.g., "How many items can you remember?"), cued-recall (e.g., "How many items that are clothing can you remember?"), and recognition-memory (e.g., "Was *apple* on the list?") conditions. Normal performance on this measure is characterized by a positive learning curve, that is, additional

---

Recall memory measures the ability to reproduce (by drawing or speaking) information that we have previously seen or heard.

Recognition memory measures our ability to identify (by answering yes or no) whether we have seen or heard something.

Free recall is the ability to remember something *freely* without any hints or help from the examiner, such as "Tell me everything you remember from the list I just read to you."

Cued recall is the ability to remember something after the examiner has given a *cue*, such as "Tell me all the things from the list that are vegetables."

An **interference condition** occurs on memory tests after the child has been asked to remember something (such as a list of objects or a story). After the child has been exposed to the original information, the examiner gives him a new list or story to remember. After this new information is provided, the child is asked to remember the original information, and the examiner evaluates how much the new information *interfered* with the child's ability to remember the information he originally learned.

items are recalled after successive learning trials. Also, performance is generally better in cued-recall than in free-recall conditions, and recognition is typically better than free recall.

Tests of Visual–Motor Abilities

Visual–motor ability is the ability to see and then do something (i.e., act using a visual–motor—either fine- or gross-motor—movement). It includes things such as the ability to see a design and copy it with a pencil. Tests of visual- motor ability can tell us about how a person is able to integrate seeing something with a motor response. Because much of learning includes the ability to integrate these two areas (e.g., copying from a blackboard), it can be an important area to assess.

The *Bender Visual Motor Gestalt Test* consists of nine cards, each displaying a simple design, such as two intersecting triangular figures. The child looks at the designs, one at a time, and copies each one on a piece of paper. Later he is asked to copy them from memory. By age twelve most children can copy the designs accurately. This is one of the most widely used visual–motor tests.

The *Developmental Test of Visual–Motor Integration (VMI)* is a test of visual–motor integration in which the child is asked to copy figures such as a circle or three-dimensional figures such as a cube, each in a single space. The test is sometimes referred to as the Beery–Buktenica Test of Visual Motor Integration, after the authors of the test.

On the *Hooper Visual Organization Test*, the child is asked to identify a picture that has been cut up into pieces and arranged in parts on the stimulus page (e.g., saw, flower). This is a test of visual perception and visual–spatial ability.

On the *Judgment of Line Orientation* test, the child is asked to judge the location and directionality of a series of lines. It is a test of spatial judgment and pure visual–spatial ability.

The *Rey–Osterrieth Complex Figure Test* is a measure of visual–motor ability, visual organization, complex constructional skills, spatial reasoning, and memory. In the test the child is asked to copy a complex geometric figure. The child's performance is scored quantitatively based on how accurately the child drew it, and, in addition, qualitative observations can be made as to the child's organizational approach. For example, the examiner can determine whether the child drew the figure in a planned manner, with good appreciation for the organizing structure or the overall organization of the design. The examiner can also assess whether the child exhibited good attention to detail. The

Rey is also used as a test of memory function, as the child is asked to re-call the figure from memory, both immediately and after a thirty-min-ute delay.

Tests of Motor Functioning

The following two tests are examples of tests that can be used to assess motor ability. As you'll notice when you read the descriptions, each test assesses how a child performs on a particular task using first the domi-nant hand (i.e., right hand for a right-handed child) and then the other, nondominant hand. The tests are useful for a few reasons. First, they provide an indication of a person's fine-motor abilities. Second, the tests can provide information regarding how well the different hemi-spheres (right or left side) of the brain are working. Because the right side of the body is controlled by the left side of the brain and the left side of the body is controlled by the right side of the brain, if a person does worse than expected with one hand than with the other (the test takes into account the dominance of one hand), the tester is given clues (along with other test data) as to whether there may be brain impair-ment. This is especially true for persons who have had a traumatic brain injury or stroke that may have affected only one side of their brains. Similarly, children with nonverbal learning disabilities, which are sometimes referred to as a "right-hemisphere disorder" (see Chap-ter Eight for more information), sometimes do worse than expected with their left hands.

On the *Finger Oscillation Task*, also known as the Finger Tapping Test, the child is asked to depress a key with her index finger (both right and left hand) as fast as she can for five trials of ten seconds each. It is a test of fine-motor speed and coordination.

The *Grooved Pegboard* test is another measure of fine-motor speed and coordination in which the child is asked to put a series of small pegs into matched holes, first with the dominant hand and then with the nondominant hand.

Tests of Executive Functions

Executive functions is a general term that includes many different abili-ties, such as organization, planning, attention, and concentration. Ex-ecutive functions are described in detail in Chapter Seven. Following are some of the more commonly used tests of executive functions.

The *Continuous Performance Test* (CPT) is a measure of sustained attentional difficulties. It measures skills such as the ability to remain vigilant, to show consistency of attentional focus, to respond quickly, and to inhibit responding. On the CPT, letters appear on a computer screen with various intervals between them. The task is to press the space bar for all letters other than the letter X.

The *Controlled Oral Word Association Test* is a test of verbal fluency that requires the child to initiate and sustain attention. On the task of letter fluency, the child is asked to rapidly generate a list of words beginning with each of three letters. On the category fluency task, the child is asked to rapidly generate a list of animals within a time limit.

The *Stroop Color and Word Test* is a formal test of impulse control in which the child is asked to read words and name colors as quickly as she can.

On the *Trail Making Test (Trails A and B)* the child is asked to "connect the dots" with numbers in Trails A and alternate between letters and numbers in Trails B. The child is timed to see how quickly he can perform this task compared with other children his age. It tests motor planning, visual attention, scanning, and the ability to "shift set" (make transitions from one thing to another).

On the *Tactual Performance Test*, the child is blindfolded and asked to fit differently shaped blocks into spaces in a board, using the dominant hand and the nondominant hand. After completing this portion of the test, the child is asked to draw the puzzle board from memory. This test assesses the child's motor speed response to an unfamiliar task and his ability to learn to use tactile and kinesthetic cues.

The *Wisconsin Card Sorting Test* (WCST) is a test in which the child is asked to sort a series of cards according to "key" cards, which vary in several elements. The child is not told how to sort the cards but rather must determine the sorting criteria. The sorting criteria shift during the test, and the individual must make decisions based only on the examiner's (or computer's) corrective feedback. It is a test of complex problem solving and abstract reasoning ability.

Projective Tests

Projective tests are measures that are used to evaluate a child's psychological or emotional functioning. Psychological functioning includes how well people manage and express their emotions, perceive the world realistically, cope with conflict, and understand themselves and their relationships and effects on others. Often the terms *psychological functioning* and *emotional functioning* are used interchangeably; however, emotional functioning is often used specifically to describe how a person is feeling (such as depressed or anxious) or how a person is managing his emotions. Projective tests are based on the assumption that individuals project their unconscious feelings and personalities when responding to ambiguous stimuli. In other words, when we are presented with a picture and asked to tell a story about it, what we say will reveal our unconscious motives and conflicts. Clinicians will often use projective testing when there is an unanswered question regarding the child's behavior or feelings about a situation. These unanswered questions can range from "Is my teenager having difficulty coping with the fact that he's adopted?" to "Is my seven-year-old experiencing some symptoms of psychosis?" to "Why is my child so anxious?" As you can see, the reasons for projective testing are broad, but in general the goal is to focus on *why* a certain behavior might be occurring.

> For example, Julie was a twelve-year-old whose parents had recently divorced. Julie appeared depressed to her mother because she didn't seem to enjoy the things she used to enjoy doing, such as sports and piano. Julie's family was in counseling, but Julie denied that she was experiencing any problems at all. In fact, she said life was "great!" The family therapist recommended projective testing to determine whether it could provide some information on why Julie's behavior (not wanting to do anything) didn't match her denial of experiencing problems. Sure enough, projective test results indicated that Julie was experiencing a lot of conflict over the fact that her parents were divorcing. She was angry at both of her parents because they appeared to be more focused on themselves and she was feeling abandoned. She felt hopeless about the future because she was afraid her parents would never stop fighting. She was sad that her mom now had to go to work and wouldn't be home with her in the afternoons anymore. The results gave the family therapist insight into Julie's world, and thus the therapist was able to direct the treatment to help Julie clarify and resolve some of these issues.

In general, projective tests require individuals to give answers to questions about vague or ambiguous stimuli, such as inkblots or pictures, or to respond to open-ended instructions such as "draw a picture of your family doing something together." Some of the more commonly used projective tests include the following:

The *Rorschach test* asks individuals to report what they see in ten different inkblots. Some of the inkblots are in black and white, and others are in color. The Rorschach is arguably the most widely used projective test and seeks to identify people's inner feelings by analyzing their interpretation of the blots. In responding to the inkblots, the person tells what he sees in each one and then reports what features in the inkblot made it look that way. Each response is scored according to formal criteria. The examiner also uses clinical judgment and one of several scoring systems to write a profile of the person's motives and conflicts. Although the Rorschach has been criticized for being too subjective and difficult to interpret, a review of studies indicates that it has moderately high validity, particularly for identifying thought disorders, or problems with thinking. In other words, people who are diagnosed as schizophrenic tend to see images that are very different from those seen by people with mild anxiety. Despite its drawbacks, the Rorschach is still considered a useful assessment tool by many clinicians, particularly when there is a question as to whether a child may have a thought disorder or psychotic thinking.

The *Thematic Apperception Test (TAT)*, *Children's Apperception Test (CAT)*, and *Roberts Apperception Test for Children (RATC)* all consist of cards containing black-and-white pictures of people in different situations. The individual is asked to tell a story about the picture, and the examiner sometimes asks follow-up questions, such as, "What events led up to the situation? How do the people in the card feel? How does the situation turn out?" The purpose of the test is to reveal a person's most important needs or conflicts. In their stories, people are thought to be expressing their own circumstances, needs, emotions, pressures, and perceptions of reality and fantasy. The psychologist looks for themes such as family conflict, aggression, and motivation.

> For example, when one of us (EB) tested Sammy, a nine-year-old who was feeling depressed, we noticed that many of his stories on the TAT included themes about absent mother figures and jealousy regarding siblings, as can be seen in the following story he told about a picture of a man and a woman working on a farm, with another woman looking off into the sunset:
>
> *One day this girl's mother and father were working in the field, and she was going to school with her Holy Bible while her parents worked. Her*

mother was pregnant, and the girl was sad that she wouldn't be the only one in the family anymore. Then the baby came, and she was happy, but later her mom died and the girl lived to be ninety-two years old.

Sammy's other stories included a high amount of conflict with his parents, particularly with his father. For example, when shown another picture of a boy looking at an open wallet on a table, Sammy told a story about a boy who steals the money and then gets "paddled" for it by his father. When we discussed these results with Sammy's mother, she indicated that, indeed, Sammy (the oldest of four children) had been feeling left out since the birth of the newest baby ten months previously. In addition, Sammy's father had been frequently absent on many business trips and had been depressed himself, often taking it out on Sammy. This type of assessment allowed us to identify one possible cause of Sammy's depression and to help pinpoint a source of underlying conflict for him.

The *sentence completion test* consists of a series of unfinished sentences that children are asked to complete, such as "School is . . . " or "If only my father would. . . . " Many versions of this test have been developed for different age groups. The test can be given orally to the child (particularly young children or those who have difficulty with writing), or it can be taken without an examiner present. We often use the test as a springboard for discussion and ask children to elaborate on their responses. The test is also useful in looking for underlying themes that are seen in other projective measures. For example, Sammy's responses on a sentence completion test reflected many of the themes he related on the TAT. When asked to respond to the sentence stem "Most mothers . . . ," he responded, "are too busy to play with their kids." When asked to complete "I sure wish my father would . . . ," Sammy responded by saying "stop hitting me."

Drawings are also sometimes used in the assessment process. The assumption is that a drawing tells us something about the person. A child's drawing can be used to corroborate themes seen in other projective tests. The more commonly used drawing tasks include the *Draw-A-Person, House–Tree–Person,* and *Kinetic Family Drawing.* On the Draw-A-Person task, the child is asked to draw a picture of a person. Once that is done, the child is asked to draw a picture of a person of the opposite gender. The House–Tree–Person task asks the child to draw separate pictures of a house, a tree, and a person. The Kinetic Family Drawing asks the child to draw a picture of his family doing something together. Other variations on these tasks include asking the child to draw a picture of a person in the rain. The clinician evaluates these drawings on the basis of emotional indicators, as well as developmental quality. For example, the developmental quality of the drawing is evaluated by determining whether children's drawings are similar in detail to that of children their own age. Emotional indicators can include things such as drawing a person who is sad or a picture of a family very disconnected from one another. Psychologists look to see if a child, when asked to draw a picture of a tree, draws a tree that looks healthy and alive. A depressed child, when asked to draw a picture of a person in the rain, might draw a picture of a person without an umbrella or shoes, dripping wet. This could be interpreted as the child feeling unprotected in his environment.

Sammy, when asked to draw a picture of a tree, drew a picture of a tree cut down to the roots. Sammy's drawing was extremely unusual, but drawings such as this should never be interpreted by themselves. However, when Sammy's drawing was viewed in light of his responses on other projective measures, it confirmed his significant depression and feelings of hopelessness.

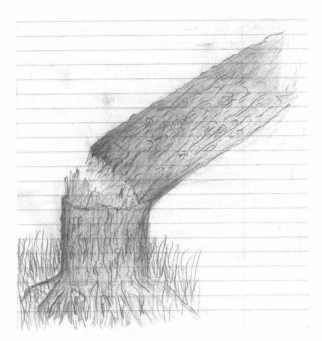

Sammy's drawing of a tree.

Self-Report and Behavioral Measures

In contrast to the subjectivity of projective measures, most self-report and behavioral measures are scored objectively, and in some cases a computer can administer and score them. These types of measures include scales, checklists, and personality inventories that can be completed by the child and/or the child's parents or teachers. The typical inventory or scale consists of a series of statements, and the child or adult is asked to indicate whether or not each statement is true for the child. There are literally hundreds of measures that would fit into this category. Some inventories measure specific areas of emotional functioning, such as anxiety, depression, and anger. Other scales measure behaviors, such as hyperactivity, inattention, and impulsivity. The scales are used to determine how far your child's behavior in a certain area is different from that of the "normal" child of roughly the same age and the same gender. For example, let's say you're worried that your five-year-old child is hyperactive. Because most five-year-olds are hyperactive at some point or another, you'll need to determine whether your child's hyperactivity is within that normal range or not. To help determine that, an evaluator will give you forms to complete that will ask you to rate your child on many different behaviors. For example, you may be asked to rate how frequently (e.g., *never, sometimes, often, almost always*) your child exhibits behaviors such as "has trouble waiting his turn," "has a short attention span," or "is easily distracted by noise." The examiner will tabulate your ratings and determine how far your child's behavior deviates from a normal five-year-old's. The examiner may also ask your child's teacher to complete similar forms so that she can compare your child's behavior at home and at school.

> In contrast to this example, Helen was a fifteen-year-old whose schoolwork had gotten considerably worse over the previous three months. She was seeing a psychiatrist who wanted to prescribe medication but who was unclear as to what extent Helen's problems were caused by anxiety or depression. The psychiatrist referred her for an evaluation, which included some measures that asked her parents and teachers to rate her behavior in many different areas. The results indicated that Helen was exhibiting significant signs of depression at home and at school, as well as significant signs of anxiety at school. Helen also completed some self-report measures that indicated that she had

many more symptoms of low self-esteem than does a typical adolescent.

As indicated earlier, there are literally countless behavioral rating scales and personality inventories. Following is a list of the more commonly used measures.

One of the most extensively researched and widely used tests of personality functioning is the *Minnesota Multiphasic Personality Inventory-2 (MMPI-2;* used for adults) and the adolescent version of this scale, the *MMPI-A.* The MMPI contains ten clinical scales, as well as a scale that can give the clinician an indication of whether it is a valid (accurate) test—that is, how open and truthful the tested child was. The ten areas measured by the test include hypochondriasis (concern with body symptoms), depression, hysteria, psychopathic deviance (disregard for social standards), masculinity/femininity (the extent to which a person has interests similar to those of the same or opposite sex), paranoia, psychasthenia (anxious, guilty feelings), schizophrenia (bizarre thoughts), hypomania (overactive, excited, impulsive), and social introversion (shy, inhibited).

The *Achenbach Child Behavior Checklist (CBCL)* has either parents or teachers rate children's behaviors in a number of different areas, such as depression, aggression, hyperactivity, and social withdrawal. The *Achenbach Youth Self-Report (YSR)* is a self-report measure for children ages, eleven to eighteen, that allows them to rate their own symptoms.

The *Behavior Assessment System for Children (BASC)* is similar to the CBCL in that it is a rating scale given to parents and teachers. However, it also includes a self-report measure for children ages eight to eighteen, as well as optional structured developmental history forms and a form for recording and classifying directly observed classroom behavior. The teacher, parent, and self-report measures yield scores on a number of different areas, including aggression, anxiety, depression, conduct problems, hyperactivity, attention problems, and withdrawal. The measures also evaluate such functioning as adaptability, leadership ability, learning problems, and social skills.

The *Children's Depression Inventory (CDI)* is a self-report measure of depression in which children indicate which phrase out of a group of phrases describes them best over the previous two weeks. It provides a measure of the presence of depressive symptoms as well as the severity of those symptoms.

Q: I've just received a copy of a neuropsychological evaluation completed with my son, David, and when I looked the tests up in this chapter, I couldn't find most of them. I don't understand what these tests were supposed to measure. Now what do I do?

A: After reading this chapter you might think that this lengthy list of tests includes nearly every potential test that might be given to your child. Unfortunately, an exhaustive brief description of tests would easily fill a 700-page book, as there are literally thousands of measures that can be used with children. We would encourage you to ask the clinician to provide you with more details about why he chose those particular tests. Because your child was supposed to have received a comprehensive evaluation, you should make sure that the clinician included measures of most, if not all, of the areas we've discussed in this chapter. Ask the clinician which of the tests measure intelligence, achievement, or language abilities, and don't be afraid to ask for more detailed information about any particular test.

Five

What Do All the Numbers Mean?

Zach's mother, Tina, was pleased with the testing. Zach seemed to enjoy the process and really liked Dr. Bagwell. Tina eagerly awaited the report. When she finally received it, she was dismayed. In it Dr. Bagwell talked about standard scores, scaled scores, *T* scores, *z* scores, and percentiles, and Tina couldn't make much sense of it as a whole. She had expected the report to clarify exactly what was wrong and why and how the test results could help Zach, but the technical terms used in the report made it really difficult for a layperson to determine whether the diagnosis was right or whether the recommendations for helping Zach were appropriate. Tina knew she needed to be able to advocate for her child, yet she had no idea whether a "standard score" of 80 in reading comprehension was good or bad. In many ways, the report left her with more questions than she had started with.

You may identify with Zach's mother. If you want to fully understand a test report, you need to know not only what the tests were meant to measure but also what the numerical scores mean. Most of the tests that were administered to Zach are called *norm-referenced* measures. In norm-referenced testing, Zach's performance is compared with the performance of a large group of participants who have taken the test. A *norm* provides an indication of what is "normal" performance. Norms are necessary because a raw test score in itself is not very meaningful. For example, suppose Zach scored 50 on a test designed to measure intelligence. What would that number mean? Even if you knew that the possible scores for this test range from 0 to 100, you wouldn't know whether 50 is what children Zach's age typically score. Fifty may be far above or below the average. If the test is to be meaningful, we have to compare Zach's performance with the performance of children who are similar (in age, grade, socioeconomic status, etc.) to Zach. It is possible to do so if the test has gone through the process of *standardization*; that is, if it has been given to a large group of children whose performance serves as the standard, or norm, against which Zach's score can be measured.

Norm-referenced tests are designed to show how well a given child performs against some average or norm.

Standardization is a procedure for establishing test norms by giving the test to large numbers of children or adults who are representative of those for whom the test is designed.

Over the years, much effort has been expended in standardizing many tests. For example, intelligence tests such as the WISC, DAS, and WAIS are administered to large groups of individuals. When we administer these tests to large numbers of children or adults of different ages, genders, ethnic backgrounds, and economic statuses selected from different parts of the United States, we find that intelligence approximates what is called a *normal distribution*. A normal distribution is sometimes called the "bell-shaped curve" because it is shaped like a bell, with the majority of scores falling in the middle of the possible range of scores and fewer scores recorded toward the extremes of the range. You can see what the normal curve looks like on the facing page.

Normal distribution or *normal curve* means the bell-shaped graph that represents the hypothetical frequency distribution for certain characteristics such as intelligence.

Many other characteristics also follow a normal curve distribution, such as height, size of vocabulary, or speed at walking a mile. On each of these dimensions, most scores would pile up in the middle, and fewer and fewer scores would occur farther away from the middle. For example, most children walk independently at twelve months. If you put this on the normal curve, you'd see that the average age for the majority of children is between ten and fourteen months, with fewer children walking at nine or fifteen months and even fewer at eight or sixteen months. The normal curve applies to an incredibly wide range of human behaviors and abilities, ranging from personality traits to motor speed to cognitive abilities and academic achievement. Most of the

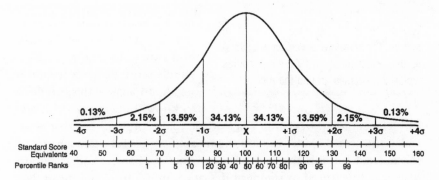

The normal curve.

behaviors assessed through testing fall along a normal distribution. One of the goals of assessment is to determine where your child's performance in a variety of areas falls on that normal curve.

This is a very important concept for two main reasons. First, many, if not most, disorders are defined by a child's behavior or performance that falls outside of the "normal" range. Second, it's important to examine the pattern of scores for each individual child to see which scores fall within the normal range and which scores fall outside the normal range. For example, a child with a math disability would likely have IQ and reading scores that fall within the average range of the normal curve but math scores that fall outside the normal range.

Explaining Performance through Test Scores

Now that you have an understanding of how scores on various tests are distributed, it should be easier to understand the various ways in which psychologists describe a person's test performance. You are likely very familiar with one of the simplest ways of describing data—the *mean*, or average. The mean is calculated by adding all scores, then dividing by the total number of scores. The mean is sometimes reported along with your child's test score. For example, eight-year-old Mitch received a score of 21.5 on the Rey–Osterrieth Complex Figure Test. In the report, we might indicate that Mitch's score is near the mean as compared with age mates. The mean is the average score for all eight-year-olds in the normative sample who have taken the Rey. In this case, the mean for eight-year-olds on the Rey is 23.64. However, comparing

The ***mean*** is the average of a set of scores. The ***standard deviation*** is a statistic that represents how far a set of scores typically disperses around the mean.

Mitch's score to the mean is not enough, because we still don't know how far the average child's score deviates from the mean. To answer this, we need to know the *standard deviation.*

The standard deviation is a statistic that represents the degree to which the scores scatter around the mean. One useful characteristic of the normal curve is that a certain percentage of scores fall at certain distances (measured in standard deviation units) from the mean. For example, about 68 percent of scores fall between plus and minus one standard deviation from the mean. About 95 percent of scores fall between plus and minus two standard deviations from the mean, and about 99 percent of scores fall between plus and minus three standard deviations from the mean. In the case of Mitch's Rey score, the standard deviation for children his age is 8 points. This means that his score falls about one-fourth of a standard deviation away from the mean and well within the average range. In general, the average range is considered to be within one to one and one-half standard deviations around the mean.

Intelligence tests generally have a mean of 100 and a standard deviation of 15. These are referred to as *standard scores.* This means that 68 percent of individuals have IQs that fall between 85 and 115 (e.g., one standard deviation above or below the mean). Similarly, 95 percent of all individuals will have IQs that fall between 70 and 130. Thus, only about 5 percent of people will have scores that fall more than two standard devia-

Standard scores have a mean of 100 and a standard deviation of 15.

tions from the mean. Because the normal curve is symmetrical, about 2.5 percent of people will score above 130, and 2.5 percent of people will score below 70. In the sidebar, you can see how children's IQ scores are classified descriptively, based on their scores.

Other tests have different means and standard deviations. For example, the subtests of most IQ tests are referred to as *scaled scores.* They are "scaled" to have a mean of 10 and a standard deviation of 3. Scholastic Assessment Tests (SAT) are normed to have a mean of 500 and a standard deviation of 100. Sometimes scores on various types of tests may be expressed in *z-scores.* The *z*-score indicates how far from the mean a person's score is, as measured in standard deviations. For ex-

Classification Ratings for the Wechsler Intelligence Scales for Children and the Wechsler Preschool and Primary Scales of Intelligence

IQ	Classification
130 and above	Very Superior
120–129	Superior
110–119	High Average
90–109	Average
80–89	Low Average
70–79	Borderline
69 and below	Mentally Deficient

ample, an IQ of 115 translates to a z-score of 1, meaning it is exactly one standard deviation above the mean. An IQ of 70 translates to a z-score of –2, meaning that it is two standard deviations below the mean.

Scores along the normal curve also represent percentiles, also known as *percentile ranks,* or the percentage of scores that fall below a particular score. People commonly confuse the terms *percentage* and *percentile,* even though they have two very different meanings. A score of 90 percent on a test means the tested person correctly answered 90 percent of the questions. When a person's score falls in the 90th percentile, it means that his score was better than the scores of 90 percent of the students who took the test. A person can get 90 percent on a test, but his score could fall at the 60th percentile, meaning that his score was better than those of only 60 percent of the students who took the test. As another way to look at this difference, you can never have a percentile rank of 100. Your score can't exceed that of 100 percent of the people tested, because you are one of them. However, you can receive a score of 100 percent on a test, meaning that you got all the answers correct. The sidebar titled "Meaning of Different IQ Scores" illustrates the meaning of different IQ scores and their relation to percentile ranks.

Take another look at the figure on page 103. Hopefully it will make clear that a child with an IQ of 100 does better than 50 percent of

Meaning of Different IQ Scores

If your IQ score is . . .	. . . then your percentile rank is . . .	Your score is higher than those in the shaded region . . .	The interpretation of your score is . . .
85	16th		Low average
100	50th		Average
115	84th		High average

same-age children (z-score of 0.0). A child with an IQ of 85 does better than 16 percent of those children (z-score of –1.0), and a child with an IQ of 130 does better than 98 percent of them (z-score of 2.0). The IQs of the vast majority of people (95.5 percent) fall between 70 and 130, with very few people receiving scores above or below those numbers.

Q: *Why are there these various ways of describing the same thing? Why can't the examiner use one way and stick to it?*

A: Unfortunately, the examiner has little latitude in reporting the scores, because the test manufacturers determine what type of scaled or standard scores are most appropriate for its tests. If your child has received a comprehensive battery, then the chances are quite high that a variety of scores will be included in the report. It would be great if all test manufacturers used the same types of scoring, but the reality is that that is very unlikely to happen.

Grade- and Age-Equivalent Scores

Many norm-referenced tests will also provide age and grade equivalents. These scores are derived by determining what the average score is for children at various ages or grade placements. For example, if the average score for twelve-year-olds on a test of reading comprehension is 50, then any child who obtains a score of 50 would receive an age-equivalent score of twelve years. In a similar way, grade-equivalent scores compare a child's score on a particular test with the average score of children at particular grade levels. A grade-equivalency score indicates the level of test performance for an average student at a certain grade level. For example, if the average score for beginning third graders on a test of spelling is 60, then a child with a score of 60 would receive a grade equivalent score of 3.0, or the beginning of third grade. Grade-equivalency scores are usually expressed in tenths of a grade (e.g., 3.5 would be mid–third grade), whereas age-equivalent scores are expressed as years and months (e.g., an age-equivalent of 10-2 would translate to ten years, two months).

Q: My child Billy was recently evaluated for ADHD. In the process of the evaluation, Billy, who is in the middle of third grade, got a grade equivalency of 7.2 in reading comprehension and 5.3 in math ability. Does this mean he should be moved up a grade?

A: Probably not. It is common for some children to perform above grade level, and performing above expectations is not considered worthy of skipping a grade. If you tested Billy's entire class, what you would find is that many children are performing at grade level, whereas some, like Billy, are performing above grade level and others are performing below. In certain public and many private school classrooms the typical child will have academic skills far above grade level. If Billy attends this type of school, his performance might be considered typical or just high average for a third grader. Similarly, just performing below grade level is not cause for retention. Instead, these scores are useful in determining a child's strengths and weaknesses, helpful in diagnosing a learning disability, and useful in devising treatment recommendations. In Billy's case, it is reassuring to know that despite difficulties with attention and concentration, he is doing quite well academically. This fact should be taken into account when developing treatment for him;

his teacher should make sure that he is challenged appropriately in the classroom. This intervention may also help address problems related to ADHD—if Billy is more engaged and challenged with the work, his attention will likely improve.

Q: *In my child's report, the doctor said the difference between her cognitive ability and her academic achievement in reading is statistically significant. What does this mean?*

A: Your child's score on an IQ test represents her cognitive ability as compared with a norm group. Similarly, her score on tests of reading represent her performance relative to children of the same age or grade level. In general, if your child receives a standard score of 115 on an IQ test, we'd expect her to receive scores around 115 on tests of reading. If her scores on reading measures are much lower than 115, we can use statistical tests to help us decide whether these differences are big enough to be meaningful. In general, scores shouldn't differ by more than one standard deviation, which in the case of standard scores would be 15 points. However, we can also look at the average difference between cognitive and academic achievement for children her age. For example, the standard deviation of the difference between cognitive ability and reading achievement might be 7 points. If your child's reading score is 14 points below her cognitive ability, it would mean that fewer than 2.5 percent of children would have that large a difference. We would call this a significant difference, meaning there is less than a 5 percent likelihood that this difference is due to chance factors.

Putting It All Together: The Report

Now that you have an idea of some of the terms used in report writing, we thought it might be helpful for you to see an actual report. This is the type of report you'd typically expect to see if you had your child evaluated at a clinic, at a hospital, or by a private psychologist. Reports from school settings will sometimes look very much like the following report and, at other times, will look quite different. School reports vary considerably from state to state and even from district to district within states.

Very often, if you've completed the evaluation through the school, you will get three or four shorter reports from the various professionals who completed the evaluations. For example, you may get one report from the school psychologist who completed the IQ test, another report from the speech and language therapist who completed the measures of language functioning, another report from the educational consultant who completed the tests of academic functioning, and another report from the occupational therapist who completed tests of motor ability. Alternatively, your school district's policy might be to have the school psychologist complete most of the testing. In that case, the report will look much like the one included here.

We've added some of our own explanations to the report to clarify. Although the report is real, the names and places mentioned in the report are not actual people or places.

The report describes a girl named Lori. Lori was referred to our clinic because her parents were confused over her teachers' concerns about her behavior. From nearly the first day of kindergarten, Lori's teachers have had concerns about her, but they have never been able to pinpoint the source. Her kindergarten teacher noticed that her handwriting was quite poor for her age and as a result made a referral to an occupational therapist, who decided that Lori could benefit from occupational therapy (OT). Lori continued to receive OT in first and second grades; however, she continued to have other problems in the classroom. For example, she wasn't making sufficient progress in reading and was placed in the lowest reading group in second grade. Furthermore, her second-grade teacher complained that she was unable to get her work done within the classroom. As her teacher noted, "When I give Lori a work sheet, she is content to just sit there and look at it for hours!"

No one could quite identify the source of Lori's problems. It didn't seem to be simply a writing or reading problem. Her teacher suspected some difficulties with attention but wasn't sure. The school was prepared to do a complete evaluation, but before it did, Lori's parents talked to their pediatrician, who recommended they get a private evaluation because a private evaluation could determine whether Lori's problems with attention were great enough to warrant a diagnosis of ADHD. If so, the evaluator could make the diagnosis (*remember, schools don't diagnose ADHD, although teacher input will be very important in making a diagnosis*) and could determine whether medication would be useful in treating the symptoms.

Lori's parents, however, also wanted the school to be invested in the evaluation process, so they requested that the school's occupational therapist and speech and language therapists complete their portion of the evaluation. This type of collaborative approach is sometimes the best of all possible worlds. Other families may make different, yet just as appropriate, decisions, which might include having the school do all of the evaluation or having the entire evaluation completed outside the school setting.

As you can see, the report is called a "Neuropsychological Evaluation," which includes tests from many areas, such as cognitive, academic achievement, and neuropsychological (remember that the term *neuropsychological tests* refers to a particular type of test that assesses neuropsychological functioning).

(*Note*: Chapter text continues on page 120.)

Neuropsychological Evaluation

PATIENT: Lori Cotter

DATE OF BIRTH: 8-3-1995

DATES OF EVALUATION: 4-16-03 and 4-30-03

AGE AT TESTING: 7 years, 8 months

Reason for Referral

Lori Cotter, a right-handed seven-year-old girl from Evergreen, MA, was referred for this evaluation to provide an assessment of her cognitive and academic functioning and rule out the possibility of attention-deficit/hyperactivity disorder. Lori's second-grade teacher has expressed concern about her writing skills in that it seems difficult and time-consuming for her to put her ideas down on paper. Last year, she received weekly occupational therapy to address fine-motor output and handwriting skills, and she will be receiving a full school-based occupational therapy evaluation shortly. While Lori's first-grade progress report indicates grade-level reading and comprehension skills, she has been placed in a lower-level reading group for second grade. Her motivation and interest in reading seem to have changed as a result because she has potentially lost confidence in herself as a reader and may not find it as pleasurable.

> The "Reason for Referral" explains why Lori needed testing. It includes the information that is most relevant to the case. The psychologist has sifted through all of the information, noted what is most pertinent, and is laying the groundwork for what is to come in the report.

> You'll notice that the evaluator has used the term *fine-motor output* here. Basically, it means trouble writing and drawing. Evaluators will often use terms that you may not understand. When in doubt, don't be afraid to ask for clarification.

Another area of concern indicated by Lori's first- and second-grade teachers is her inability to focus consistently on her work, particularly now that she is in second grade. The ability to work independently, organizational skills, time-management skills, concentration, and effort were all rated as "needs improvement" on her latest progress report from school. At home, Lori's parents notice that she is somewhat disorganized (e.g., she has a very messy room) and has to be coaxed into do-

> When an evaluator uses the term *rule out*, it means that someone, such as a doctor or teacher, has wondered whether Lori may have ADHD, and as a result the evaluator will determine whether the diagnosis is appropriate. It might seem that a more appropriate term would be to rule *in* the diagnosis of ADHD. This term is used, though, because psychologists work with the assumption that the child does *not* have a diagnosable problem. As a result, they are looking for evidence that the diagnosis can be confirmed.

> *Decoding* is the ability to sound out words. As we've said before, expect the report to include some terms you may not be familiar with. Don't hesitate to ask for clarification.

ing her homework. Her parents' observations of Lori's reading skills contrast with those of the teacher, because she seems to decode and understand grade-level text with relative ease.

Lori attends the Eisenhower Elementary School, which is part of the Evergreen School District. She is in a regular-education second-grade class with nineteen students and one teacher. She does not receive any formal special education services but gets reading assistance in a group format. In addition to the OT evaluation she will be receiving soon at school, Lori will undergo a full speech and language evaluation there.

Lori lives at home with her parents and older brother. Her developmental and medical histories are without major concern, though she presents with heightened sensitivity to odors and touch and has asthma that is treated with inhalers as needed.

Evaluation Procedures

- Interview with mother
- Developmental Intake Form
- Review of records
- Behavior Assessment System for Children (BASC)–Parent and Teacher Forms
- ADHD Rating Scale
- Wechsler Intelligence Scale for Children–Third Edition (WISC-III)
- Wechsler Individual Achievement Test–Second Edition (WIAT-II)
- Test of Written Language (TOWL-3) Story Writing test
- Developmental Test of Visual–Motor Integration (VMI)
- Rey–Osterrieth Complex Figure Test
- WRAML Sentence Memory and Story Memory subtests
- Trail Making Test, Trails A and B
- Stroop Color and Word Test
- Wisconsin Card Sorting Test (WCST)
- Grooved Pegboard Test

Behavioral Observations

Lori presented as a friendly, cooperative person who seemed invested in performing her best on the various tests given. She established and maintained effective eye contact and responded well to the evalua-

> *Behavioral observations* include things that the psychologist observed about your child during the testing session. Expect the examiner to comment on things such as your child's appearance, interpersonal skills, speech and language, attitude toward the testing (e.g., positive or negative), motor activity (e.g., hyperactive, underactive), motivation, emotions and mood, attention, and persistence.

tor's attempts to engage her. Lori initiated conversation at appropriate times throughout the sessions and demonstrated a good sense of humor. She sustained effort well, even on more challenging tasks.

In this quiet setting, Lori focused well and was not overly distractible. She remained seated easily and was not excessively fidgety or restless. At times, she responded impulsively and made "careless"/impulsive errors (e.g., she did not attend to the operation sign on the math work sheet and therefore added rather than subtracted—though correctly). This was not found to occur with enough frequency or severity to have significantly affected her test scores, however.

In general, the following results were found to provide a valid estimate of Lori's current cognitive and academic functioning as assessed under structured conditions.

Test Results

General Intellectual Functioning

On the WISC-III, Lori obtained a Verbal IQ score of 129 (97th percentile), which is in the Superior range. Her Performance IQ score was 106 (66th percentile), which is in the Average range. Because of the statistically significant difference between these scores (23 points), Lori's resulting Full Scale IQ score of 121 (92nd percentile, Superior range) should be interpreted with caution. In light of her history of fine-motor

> Lori's Verbal IQ score at the 97th percentile means she scored better than 97 out of 100 children in this area.

output concerns and observed motor-planning issues, Lori's Verbal IQ score, in the Superior range, was determined to provide the more accurate estimate of her intelligence level and was used in comparison with subsequent test scores to determine areas of relative strength and weakness.

Lori's index scores were as follows: Verbal Comprehension—134 (99th percentile); Perceptual Organization—114 (82nd percentile); Freedom from Distractibility—104 (61st percentile); and Processing Speed—77* and 93 (6th and 32nd percentiles, respectively). (See page 105 for an explanation of percentiles and percentages.) In comparison with her estimated Superior intelligence level, the latter two scores were found to reflect potential areas of relative weakness for Lori.

> In the preceding sentence, the examiner has listed areas that are weaknesses for Lori. Examiners will generally do this if weaknesses or strengths can be noted.

Lori's individual subtest scores are presented below. Scores of 4 and 5 are borderline deficient; 6 to 8 are low average; 9 to 11 are average; 12 and 13 are high average; 14 and 15 are superior; and 16 to 19 are very superior.

Many examiners will clarify scores in this way; however, some won't. When in doubt, ask your examiner what they mean.

Verbal Subtests	Scaled Scores	Performance Subtests	Scaled Scores
Information	16	Picture Completion	14
Similarities	14	Coding	5
Arithmetic	11	Picture Arrangement	12
Vocabulary	18	Block Design	13
Comprehension	16	Object Assembly	10
(Digit Span)	(10)	(Symbol Search)*	(6/12)

*Subtest was readministered during the second appointment as Lori lost the task set on the first trial.

A "loss of task set" means that a child forgot what she was supposed to be doing.

Lori's scores varied greatly, with a range from 5 (borderline deficient) to 18 (very superior). While a somewhat uneven profile is not that unusual for younger children such as Lori, the extent of the variability suggests specific areas of strength and weakness. In general, Lori's fine-motor output and fine-motor planning difficulties were the most prominent areas of concern and significantly affected her overall Performance IQ score (coding and object assembly scores). Another area that was found to be less developed than would be predicted based on Lori's estimated superior intelligence level is her capacity to maintain information in working memory and manipulate it (Arithmetic; Digit-Span-reversed). These scores were average, however, indicating generally age-appropriate skill but a potential weakness relative to her other abilities.

In this paragraph, the examiner is describing Lori's performances on specific tests and how they relate to one another and to the overall IQ scores. Fine-motor output and fine-motor planning, areas of difficulty for Lori, include the ability to write quickly, as well the ability to organize one's approach to written work.

Achievement/Academic Functioning

On the WIAT-II, Lori obtained the following scores (SS = Standard Score; percentile = percentile; GE = Grade Equivalent.)

Remember that Standard Scores generally have a mean of 100 and a standard deviation of 15.

Neuropsychological Evaluation *(cont.)*

Subtest	SS	Percentile	GE
Word Reading	110	75	3:0
Pseudoword Reading	109	73	3:0
Reading Comprehension	114	83	3:0
Spelling	105	63	2:5
Written Expression	111	77	3:0
Math Reasoning	110	75	3:1
Numerical Operations	102	55	2:5

TOWL-3 Story Writing: Contextual Conventions
Scaled Score = 12 (75th percentile)

Contextual Language Scaled Score = 11 (63rd percentile)

Story Construction Scales Score = 10 (50th percentile)

> Scaled scores have a mean of 10 and a standard deviation of 3.

Based on these results, Lori was found to be capable of achieving on or above her current grade level (2:5) in all of the academic areas assessed. Her scores were not significantly below those predicted using the WISC–WIAT discrepancy criteria. She was found to be strongest in her reading comprehension skills, which were found to be in the high average range and advanced by half a grade level.

Lori's written expression skills were also found to be on or somewhat above her current grade level at the one-word-, sentence-, and paragraph-length levels. When combining sentences, Lori consistently used *and* in order to do so, which detracted from the quality of her writing but is typical of the mid-second grader. On the TOWL-3 Story Writing task, Lori needed encouragement to continue working after completing two sentences about a space scene ("There is a spaceship blasting off. There is a guy on the moon"), which she did in 107 seconds. She then added, "There is a sadalite. A guy deayes," which required another 88 seconds. She therefore completed a four-sentence paragraph in 3'15".

Lori's writing performance was notable for graphomotor and motor-planning issues in that words were often spaced too closely together, letter size was variable, and the gaps between words were irregular. She also

> Are you picking up on a pattern here? Several times, the examiner has highlighted Lori's problems with motor planning, graphomotor weaknesses, and fine-motor difficulties. As such, the examiner is building a case that services are needed in this area.

tended to make "careless" mistakes, likely out of haste, which affected her spelling (e.g., when copying from two printed sentences, she wrote, "The frog is geen and jups," though she did go back and add the *m* in *jumps*.)

Visual–Motor/Spatial Skills

On the VMI, a structured test of visual–motor integration skills, Lori obtained a standard score of 94 (34th percentile), which is in the average range and has an age equivalent of 6 years, 11 months. This score represents an area of relative weakness in comparison with Lori's estimated intelligence level.

On the Rey–Osterrieth Complex Figure, a test of visual–motor integration, constructional skills, and organization, Lori obtained a Copy score of 16, which is average for her age. While she initially copied the perimeter of the figure as an effective first step organizationally, Lori then had difficulty managing the complexity of the interior details. Likely as a result, her Delayed Recall score after thirty minutes fell to 1, which is in the low-average to borderline-deficient range for her age.

On the WISC-III subtests that rely heavily on spatial skills, Lori performed better on the task that required more analytic skills (Block Design) than organizational/synthesis skills (Object Assembly).

> You'll notice that there is a reference to the WISC here. Because intelligence tests such as the WISC tap multiple areas, a child's performance on the WISC will often be mentioned at different points in the report where it is relevant.

Executive Functions

With regard to Lori's capacity for sustained auditory attention, her skills varied somewhat but were generally in the low-average to average range (WISC-III Arithmetic and Digit Span; WRAML Sentence Memory scaled score = 8; WRAML Story Memory scaled score = 9). It should be noted that Lori's delayed-recall score on the Story Memory test increased by three points as she recalled five more details on one of the stories after a thirty-minute delay; this suggests that she actually attended to the information better than one would assume from her score but had difficulty with its immediate recall. On measures that relied heavily on sustained visual attention,

> *Executive functions* include tasks that measure the ability to plan and be flexible in one's plans, to organize one's behaviors, to monitor one's performance, and to inhibit the impulse to respond, as well as working memory.

Lori scored generally in the high-average to superior range (WISC-III Picture Arrangement and Picture Completion), suggesting that she attends more effectively to information that is presented visually.

On the Stroop, a measure of impulse control and sustained concentration, Lori's scores were in the average range (50th to 58th percentiles). On

Trails A, a basic sequencing and visual scanning test, Lori scored in the average range for speed, and she did not make any errors. On Trails B, a test of complex sequencing, scanning, and shifting set, Lori experienced difficulty. She had trouble maintaining the task demand and made four errors; her test score was subsequently low-average range. A similar finding emerged on the WCST, as Lori scored below the first percentile in maintaining set, or keeping the task demand in working memory. This score was in stark contrast to all the others on this measure, which were in the average to superior range, indicating effective complex problem-solving and reasoning skills. Finally, organizational difficulties were observed on a visual–spatial task (Rey–Osterrieth) and subsequently affected the retention and recall of the information over time. General organizational difficulties were noted and reported by her parents and current teacher.

Sensorimotor Processing

On the Grooved Pegboard, Lori completed the short-form version in an average of 32.5 seconds with her dominant (right) hand and did not drop any pegs; this score is average for her age. However, Lori needed to be reminded to work from right to left, even after two practices. Using her left hand, she completed the test in an average of 44.5 seconds, which is average for her age.

Behavioral Functioning

Lori's mother and teacher completed the ADHD Rating Scale and the Behavior Assessment System for Children (BASC). Their ratings were quite similar, with ratings on the BASC Attention Problems scale falling in the clinically significant range. They reported that Lori often daydreams or is easily distracted and unable to concentrate. Lori's teacher indicated that Lori "really wants to please but needs constant help at refocusing." Lori's teacher indicated that Lori's attentional difficulties impact her school performance. Their ratings on the ADHD Rating Scale were also quite similar and consistent with a diagnosis of ADHD, predominantly inattentive type.

Diagnostic Impressions

Attention-Deficit/Hyperactivity Disorder, Predominantly Inattentive Type, 314.00

> The numbers that follow the diagnosis correspond to the *Diagnostic and Statistical Manual* diagnostic coding.

Summary and Recommendations

Lori Cotter is a seven-year-old girl in the second grade who was found to have an estimated Superior intelligence level, though it should be noted that a 23-point difference between her Verbal (higher) and Performance

scores was found. This difference was attributed to Lori's history of difficulty with fine-motor output and observed motor-planning issues, which
negatively affected two test scores in particular. This finding was in no way
found to indicate the presence of a nonverbal learning disorder due to the
lack of additional criteria necessary for this diagnosis to be made (e.g.,
problems with social skills, gross-motor development, sensory integration,
or significant problems with math and reading comprehension).

You should expect the summary to
provide a short recap of the test results. It should give you a snapshot
of the important findings, as well as a
diagnosis, if a diagnosis is indicated.

Achievement testing indicated that
Lori is capable of on- or above-grade,
level work in all of the academic are as
assessed, including areas thought to be
potential weaknesses by the school
(e.g., reading comprehension and written expression). Perhaps her teacher
has realized how bright Lori is and has found that other skills, writing in particular, do not seem to come as easily to her as one would expect. Nevertheless, her skills were determined to be within the expected range, given her estimated intelligence level, age, and grade level.

Lori's performance on a number of measures of executive functions, as
well as behavioral rating scales, supports a diagnosis of ADHD, Predominantly Inattentive Type. In the executive function domain, Lori's capacity for
sustained auditory attention, working memory, and maintaining set were
found to be potential weaknesses. Organizational concerns were noted but
were found to be isolated with respect to visual–spatial/motor functioning.

Based on the information acquired in the evaluation, the following
recommendations are made:

Recommendations should be specific
and easy to understand and implement. Keep in mind, though, that just
because an independent evaluator
recommends something, the school
district is not required to implement it.

1. While this evaluator defers to the
   recommendations made by the
   school occupational therapist regarding the specific treatment
   goals and strategies, the results obtained here support the need for continued individual occupational therapy to address graphomotor skills,
   fine-motor planning, motor-output speed, fine-motor processing, and
   strength. Visual organizational skills should also be emphasized. The OT
   should consult with Lori's teacher to implement any classroom accommodations or strategies for increasing her functioning in these areas.
2. To assist Lori in maintaining set, or retaining task instructions, she
   should be provided with written and verbal directions to tests and assignments. It may also be helpful to provide prompts if she seems to
   be getting off task or appears lost.
3. To maximize Lori's focus in class, these strategies are recommended:
   a. Preferential seating

  b. Use multisensory, especially hands-on, instruction methods—at least always pair verbal information with visual aids

  c. Work in small groups

  d. Provide external structure for more open-ended tasks

  e. Give only brief, one-step instructions

  f. Give her extra time to proof her work

  g. Break tasks up into their smaller components

  h. Allow for brief breaks throughout the day

4. Although Lori performed within expected time limits during this evaluation, the teacher's report indicates that she often runs out of time when doing written work. She should then be provided with extra time to complete written assignments, with time notices as she goes along (e.g., every five minutes and especially when she has only five minutes left). Her relatively slow processing speed as noted in the WISC-III results also supports the recommendation for extra time on tests and in-class assignments.

> If you find that your school is unable to provide services, you may want to contact an advocate who can help advocate within the school on your child's behalf.

5. To facilitate Lori's ability to put her ideas into writing, she should receive keyboarding instruction if she is not already able to type well. The use of a computer/word processor for writing assignments may prove helpful in this way.

6. The results of this evaluation and parent report support the recommendation to remove Lori from her current reading group. This will likely enhance her confidence around reading assignments and will allow her to be appropriately challenged with reading activities.

7. Confidence seems to be an issue with Lori's writing skills as well; thus, it is important that her parents and teachers support her without conveying a sense that she is somehow not capable enough in this area, as test results show she truly is.

8. To ensure Lori's confidence around academics, it may be fun and helpful for her to serve as a peer tutor or mentor to a younger student in reading, vocabulary skills, etc.

9. A psychopharmacological evaluation should be pursued to determine if stimulant medication would be helpful for Lori's symptoms of ADHD.

> Lori's school district, upon receipt of this report, as well as findings from their occupational and speech therapist, decided to place Lori on an IEP. Had she needed only accommodations and not direct services (i.e., occupational therapy), her needs could likely have been met with a 504 Plan.

  It was a pleasure to work with Lori. Given her parents' permission, I would be available to discuss the results of this evaluation.

XXXXX XXXXX, PhD
Licensed Clinical Psychologist

Lori's mother was very pleased with the report and the results of the testing. She felt the report really put things together for her. She finally had an explanation for why Lori behaved the way she did. It turned out that Lori had extremely good verbal skills and grade-appropriate academic skills, which explained why she was progressing well—a great relief to her mother. But Lori also had slow processing speed—meaning that it takes her longer to do certain types of work, such as work sheets, than it does other children—and she has trouble with written output and difficulty concentrating. These difficulties are causing her to have significant problems in the classroom despite her high intelligence.

After the evaluation, Lori's parents decided to pursue a number of the recommendations suggested in the report. First, as mentioned earlier, Lori's school placed her on an IEP, which entitled her to special services such as occupational therapy, extra time on tests, and extra help with organizing her work. Second, Lori's parents decided to seek a psychopharmacological evaluation with a child psychiatrist to determine whether medication would be helpful in treating her symptoms of inattention. The psychiatrist recommended trying Concerta, a stimulant medication used to treat symptoms of ADHD. The effect on Lori's performance in the classroom was remarkable. By year's end, Lori had, according to her teacher, "gone from the bottom of the class to the top of the class."

Psychopharmacology is a field within psychiatry that includes professionals who specialize in the administration of psychiatric medications.

Lori's parents were pleased that the evaluation process had resulted in changes in Lori's educational environment and behavior. Although we can't promise results like this for every child, the evaluation should provide you with some answers as to *why* your child is having problems, *what* effect the problems might have on the child's day-to-day functioning, and *how* to remedy those problem areas.

Part III

Common Childhood Disorders

Six

Dyslexia

Dyslexia is the most common of all of the known learning disabilities, affecting one out of five children in the United States and accounting for 80 percent of those diagnosed with a learning disability. It affects boys and girls equally and is lifelong, not something that a person outgrows. This reading disorder, which is sometimes referred to as *developmental dyslexia,* is characterized by difficulty in learning to read and spell despite conventional instruction and adequate intelligence. It is neurologically based and often familial; that is, it tends to run in families, which suggests that it is genetically founded and inherited. People can acquire dyslexia through factors that cause neurological disturbance, but it is not caused by poor eyesight, poor hearing, inadequate teaching or schooling, ethnic background, or economic level.

Most people who are dyslexic are born with the disorder, but the vast majority are not diagnosed until they've reached reading age. The reason is that diagnosis involves determining whether a child's ability to read and spell is substantially less than would be expected based on her age, intelligence, and educational level. Diagnosis is accomplished through standardized, individually administered tests of intelligence, academic achievement, and cognitive processing. These can include tests of language, memory, and executive functions useful in identifying the most effective treatments for the child's specific problems.

Most researchers and educators now agree that children with dyslexia have difficulty with reading and related skills, such as spelling, reading comprehension, and writ-

The terms *dyslexia* and *reading disorder* are often used interchangeably. The simplest definition of either is a significant unexpected difficulty in learning to read or spell.

Phonological skills are the abilities involved in understanding the rules by which sounds go with letters, also known as *grapheme–phoneme correspondence* (letter–sound correspondence).

ing, because of problems with phonological processing. Phonological processing involves the ability to accurately perceive the distinct sounds that make up a word; these individual sounds are referred to as *phonemes*. For example, when you are learning to read the word *cat,* you need to be able to segment the word into its separate phonemes—"cuh," "aah," and "tuh." You then need to blend these sounds together to form the word *cat.* Most children with dyslexia have difficulty perceiving the individual sounds or phonemes in words and therefore have trouble with the task of breaking words down to sound them out for reading or spelling.

> Remember Philip, the fourth grader who had had few school problems previously but who was currently struggling with reading assignments and homework? He was referred for testing even though up until the present he had performed about on grade level in his work. When Philip's mother was interviewed by the evaluator, she recalled, in looking back, that he did not seem to learn his letters nearly as easily as his older siblings had. He also needed a lot more practice learning the sounds that the letters made—letter–sound correspondence. She recalled that he had often mixed up letters that looked similar, such as *b* and *d,* as he could not remember which one made which sound. Philip's spelling had "always been a problem," according to his mother, and now that he was being asked to read more difficult material and write about it, he was having a lot of trouble.
>
> Philip was first tested through the public schools. He was found to be of high-average intelligence, but his word decoding skills—his ability to sound out words—were at about the third-grade level, one year or so behind. It was not surprising to find that Philip's spelling skills were even more delayed, because spelling requires the same phonetic decoding skills that reading does. On a test of reading comprehension, Philip performed below grade level again. He was noted to make many errors in reading that then interfered with his ability to make sense of what had been written. Instead of reading the sentence "The dog was now inside the house," Philip read, "The dog was *not* inside the house," which changed his understanding of what had actually happened in the story. Because of many spelling and organizational problems, Philip's creative writing skills were also found to be at least one year below grade level.

Although the school psychologist documented all of these skill delays and recommended reading and writing support once a week, Philip's parents were dissatisfied with the lack of an explanation for why Philip was having these problems now. Philip was evaluated privately and was diagnosed with dyslexia. In addition to the type of testing that the school system did, Philip received tests of phonological processing that helped determine why he was having so much trouble reading. These tests showed that Philip had not mastered the decoding skills that would otherwise allow him to read the new and more difficult words that were showing up in his fourth-grade textbooks. He had been able to memorize the appearance of many common words, which had helped him get by up until the present. In fourth grade, however, the work became significantly harder, and students were asked to do a lot more work on their own. In second and third grade, the class read aloud together, which also helped Philip "read" his assignments. Now that he had to do most of the work by himself, he was really struggling.

The clinical psychologist who evaluated Philip privately was able to make the diagnosis of dyslexia and provided appropriate recommendations for Philip. The school system agreed to provide the recommended services given that the diagnosis of dyslexia had been made with thorough documentation of Philip's delays. After a year of intensive instruction in Wilson Reading, one of the multisensory reading methods, Philip's decoding skills were slightly above grade level. He continues to receive special education services and accommodations for his writing and organizational skills, including direct instruction and extra time to complete in-class assignments and tests. Spelling remains an area of difficulty for Philip, and he uses a spell-check device to assist him in his written work, as well as learning special spelling rules and strategies. On tests, his teachers do not penalize him for spelling errors. Philip's parents were advised to have him reevaluated in two to three years to assess his progress and amend his educational program as needed.

Q: I've been concerned about my first grader's reading skills, especially since her older siblings were reading short books by her age. When I expressed my concerns to her teacher, he said, "Don't worry–she's just a late bloomer. She'll catch up to the class over time." I'm not comfortable just waiting, but I don't want to seem like a "never satisfied" parent. What should I do?

A: What you have just described seems to happen often with students with dyslexia. For a variety of reasons, but usually financial, schools do not like to initiate the evaluation of students who seem to be lagging slightly behind their peers, especially in the early grades, as with your child. Because children learn at variable rates, and because the ages of children in a given class can vary, there are cases of particular students who do catch on a bit later than their classmates yet experience no difficulties in the future. However, your intuition, as well as your experience raising children who have learned to read already, are telling you that something seems wrong with your first grader.

The good news is that even without the support of your child's teacher, you have the legal right to request a full evaluation funded by the school and performed by appropriate school staff (usually the school psychologist, special education teachers, speech and language therapist, and occupational therapist if need be). To start this evaluation process, referred to as a "team evaluation," you must put the request and the reason for it in writing and send it to the director of special education for your child's school system. We also recommend sending a copy to the teacher and the principal of the school to keep them informed and to alert them to your concerns.

Once your letter is received, the school must complete your child's evaluation in a reasonable period of time; check your state law, as some states set a specific time period (e.g., thirty days) in which the school must finish the testing. You should be contacted for information during the evaluation period, and you should be asked to attend a team meeting at the end of the evaluation to review the results and to discuss recommendations for services. If the school's testing found that your child has significant delays in reading and spelling skills relative to grade and/or intelligence level, the team is likely to recommend that your child receive special education services for these skills. The frequency and intensity of the services varies depending on the severity of the problem and, frankly, on the quality and resources of the school system. Prior to the team meeting, you are encouraged to learn about your rights to contest the school's educational plan for your child should you feel that the school has missed the problem or is not addressing it appropriately. See Chapters 2 and 3 for more information on getting an evaluation from the school system.

Diagnosing Dyslexia

What the Testing Evaluation Should Include

As Philip's case demonstrates, tests of reading and spelling are necessary to confirm a diagnosis of dyslexia. However, a thorough evaluation will include, at a minimum:

- An interview with the parent and child (typically done separately) that includes information about the child's family history, school history, and reading and language history
- Screening for common coexisting conditions, such as attention-deficit/hyperactivity disorder
- Tests, including:
  - Intelligence tests (see Chapter Four)
  - Multiple measures of reading and spelling, including measures of decoding, nonword reading, oral reading, and reading comprehension (described later)
  - Tests of mathematical ability and other areas of academic achievement
  - Neuropsychological tests, including measures of language processing abilities, visual–spatial abilities, attention, and memory (see Chapter Four)

It is important that the person doing the evaluation be a licensed professional who has experience in testing for dyslexia. The evaluator should also be trained in other learning disabilities and psychological issues, because it will be this person's job to determine which diagnosis (if any) is most appropriate for your child. The evaluation we have described is most often done by a licensed psychologist or neuropsychologist. Experienced professionals may be independent practitioners and/ or affiliated with a clinic, university, or teaching hospital. Pediatric neurologists and developmental pediatricians are also often involved in the diagnostic process. Although school psychologists are extremely important members of a child's treatment team, they are not always the best people to assess the child for dyslexia, because schools do not diagnose psychiatric disorders and learning disabilities. Instead, their focus is on determining areas of skill weaknesses and appropriate placement and services.

Once a diagnosis of dyslexia has been made, we recommend that children be reassessed every two to three years to make sure they are making expected progress. The assessment may often include only the area of reading. If your child is on an IEP, the school is required to perform an assessment during this time frame. However, testing should be undertaken sooner if your child is experiencing increased difficulties.

Preparing for a Dyslexia Evaluation

Be prepared for a typical dyslexia evaluation to take four to six hours. Most psychologists will either schedule one long testing session or divide the time up into two or three shorter test sessions. There are pros and cons to doing either one long or two or three shorter sessions. Scheduling an evaluation over more than one time slot means that the child doesn't have to concentrate for a lengthy time period but also means that the child has to be taken out of school for more than one day.

We both typically do our evaluations in one lengthy session. Many times parents will tell us when they book their child's appointment that their child will *never* be able to concentrate for that long. However, we almost never find that is the case. One benefit to doing a longer test session is that it gives us the opportunity to see how the child reacts both when at his best and when more fatigued. It gives a sense of what the child is like in the normal classroom setting, in which he is required to concentrate for a much longer day. We generally leave the less challenging tests until the end of the session and complete the more challenging ones near the beginning of the session. We also take frequent breaks for lunch or snacks.

If we make an appointment with parents who are very concerned about the length of testing, we generally ask them to make one appointment with the option of coming back if we can't get through everything. Our primary goal is to get the most valid evaluation of that child. There is no right or wrong way to schedule an evaluation as long as the psychologist is comfortable with the procedure and the child's testing is valid as a result of the process.

You may be wondering how you can prepare your child for this type of evaluation. First, let your child know you are pursuing this evaluation because you want to know how she learns best. Depending on your child's age, you may be able to be open with the child, saying something like, "I know you've been struggling in school lately, and I want to find out how to make things better for you." Second, talk to your child about what to expect. Explain that the child will be spending a few hours with someone doing a variety of things—puzzles, solving problems, drawing, defining words, math, reading, spelling, writing— and that many kids have an evaluation just like this at one time or another. Also let your child know that most kids really like being tested! This may be hard to believe, but it's true. Most kids find the process rather fun. Even though some of the tests may be difficult, a good evaluator will keep the process upbeat and never let a child feel absolutely discouraged. As a result, kids usually enjoy the process.

Unfortunately, this type of evaluation is not typically covered by most insurance companies, and as a result you'll likely be paying out of pocket. A typical comprehensive evaluation can cost anywhere from $1,200 to $2,500 (or more, depending on where you live). Your child can receive testing through your local school district; however, the school will not be able to give your child a diagnosis of dyslexia. If a diagnosis is important, you'll need to have an independent evaluation. For more information on getting an independent evaluation, see Chapter Two.

Commonly Used Tests of Reading Ability

Measures of Single-Word Reading

A number of measures of single-word reading (the ability to read words presented to a child one at a time) are commonly used in testing for dyslexia, and they are all quite similar. They are used to measure how well the child can decode (read aloud) words. The tests typically require the child to recognize and name letters and pronounce words. The most frequently administered tests (previously described in Chapter Four) are:

- Wechsler Individual Achievement Tests: Basic Reading subtest.
- Differential Ability Scales: Reading subtest. Typically used if the examiner has measured intelligence using the DAS.
- Woodcock–Johnson Psycho-Educational Battery–Revised: Letter–Word Identification subtest.
- Wide Range Achievement Test 3: Reading subtest

Other tests of reading include:

Woodcock–Johnson Word Attack Subtest

This subtest asks the child to read words that are not real words, such as *grep* or *untriokest*. It is a very important test in diagnosing dyslexia because children must rely solely on their phonological decoding skills, having never seen or heard these letter strings before. Therefore, intelligent children with dyslexia may perform within the normal range on tests of single-word reading (because they have been able to memorize the words by sight) but may have much difficulty on a test of nonword reading. A dyslexia assessment should typically include a test of word attack or pseudoword decoding.

Gray Oral Reading Test (GORT-IV)

The GORT-IV is a timed reading test that requires the child to read passages out loud. The examiner records the length of time it takes the child to read the passages and also records the number and types of errors the child makes. The examiner then asks the child questions about what he has read. The test yields three scores: rate (how quickly the child read the passage), accuracy (how accurately the child read the passage), and comprehension (how well the child understood what he read). It is a very useful test in diagnosing dyslexia because it is a timed test, and it is often a better indicator of actual school performance than tests of single-word reading (which do not have a time limit) because unlimited time is rarely available in the classroom.

Gates–MacGinitie Reading Tests

The Gates is a paper-and-pencil multiple-choice test that comes in three grade and high school levels. The tests measure two aspects of reading. On the vocabulary subtest, the individual reads a word silently and is then asked to determine which of several choices is its synonym. On the comprehension subtest, the individual reads a series of passages silently and then answers written multiple-choice questions about their meaning.

Lindamood Test of Auditory Conceptualization

A test of phoneme awareness and segmentation skills (which are important skills underlying reading ability), this test requires the child to represent sounds with colored blocks and then manipulate those blocks as the order of the sounds heard is changed. So, for example, a child might choose a red and yellow block to represent the two sounds (phonemes) in *pa*. The child is then asked to manipulate the colored blocks to represent *ap* and, in a more complex task, *pap*. The ability to recognize sounds and to sequence these sounds is important to progress in reading and spelling.

Tests of Reading Comprehension

Tests of reading comprehension evaluate how well a child understands what she has read. These tests can vary widely. Some are timed (such as the Gates), and some are untimed. Some ask the child to read a lengthy passage, and others ask the child to read a sentence or two. In addition to those mentioned, other commonly used tests of reading comprehension include:

- WIAT Reading Comprehension subtest: This tests asks the child to read a short passage and answer a question about what he has read. There is no time limit.
- Nelson–Denny Reading Test: This test is very similar to the Gates in that it provides a measure of vocabulary and comprehension. It has a time limit.

Q: So if my child has dyslexia, will he perform poorly on all of these tests?

A: Not necessarily. Variability is common in people with and without dyslexia. What is most often seen in children with dyslexia is that the areas that require phonics skills are the weakest. Children with dyslexia tend to score lower on tests of spelling, timed oral reading, and nonword reading, in comparison with general intellectual skills. Children with dyslexia can often show much better reading comprehension, because language competence (as opposed to reading competence) contributes significantly to good performance on this test. Reading comprehension is also highly correlated with verbal IQ, particularly in children with reading difficulties. A child who has a high verbal IQ may perform quite well on a comprehension test but still be dyslexic. Performance on the GORT-IV test will often differ from that on the reading subscales of the Woodcock–Johnson or WIAT because the GORT-IV provides a timed measure of reading fluency and speed, rather than comprehension or word recognition, which are often given unlimited time.

Q: *My child is in first grade and can't read a word. He is undergoing an evaluation for dyslexia. These tests you've mentioned don't seem to fit for him. Are there other tests of reading that are used for younger children?*

A: Yes, there are tests of reading that are used for younger children (typically ages four to six). These include:

- *Lindamood Test of Auditory Conceptualization*: See the preceding description.
- *Rosner Test of Auditory Analysis Skills*: This tests the important skill of phoneme segmentation. The examiner tells the child: "Say 'meat.' " The child is then asked to "Say 'meat' again but don't say the 'm.' " Another example is "Say 'smack' now say it again, but don't say 'm.' " The inability to do this is highly related to dyslexia.
- *Slosson Test of Reading Readiness*: This tests the ability to identify letters, to rhyme, to sequence a story, and to visually discriminate. It can be used with children ages four to seven.
- *Gates–MacGinitie Reading Test*: The Pre- and Readiness Levels of this test look at awareness of prereading skills, such as identification of print, identification of letters, and identification of letter–sound correspondences.
- *Roswell–Chall Diagnostic Reading Test of Word Analysis Skills*: This test breaks down different aspects of the decoding process to see what specific rules the child does or does not know, such as consonant sounds, consonant digraphs, vowel sounds, and the rule of the silent *e*.

Q: *My two older children have dyslexia, and I strongly suspect that I do, too. I am worried about my other child, who is four, and want to know how early you can tell whether someone has dyslexia.*

A: Given the increased risk of dyslexia in children whose parents are also affected, you are right to be concerned. The latest research has shown that a child with one dyslexic parent will have a 23 to 65 percent chance of also having the disorder; this risk goes up if both parents are dyslexic. The rate of dyslexia in children with only one affected parent is five to seven times the risk for children born to nondyslexic parents. In addition, a sibling of a child who is dyslexic has a 40 percent chance of also having the disorder.

Although unfortunately most children with dyslexia are not diagnosed until third grade, it is possible to note early red flags in three- and four-year-olds and to formally diagnose dyslexia in children as young as five. The early warning signs for dyslexia include a family history of the disorder, language delays, difficulty rhyming, problems learning or remembering frequently heard children's songs, confusing words that sound alike, and problems with word retrieval (difficulty coming up with the name of frequently used items, etc.). Other red flags include difficulty learning the letters of the alphabet, problems learning the sounds that go with the letters, trouble saying the sounds that make up a word (which most children can do by age four), and a limited expressive vocabulary (they do not use a lot of different words to communicate).

Given your family history, we would recommend having your four-year-old child formally tested at age five. In the meantime, however, we suggest you try fun activities that will likely promote your child's reading skills, regardless of whether he has dyslexia. Reading with your child is always beneficial—at least a half hour a day, but more if you can. Using children's books that contain a lot of rhyming and a variety of sounds, such as Dr. Seuss books, is especially recommended. You might also play rhyming games, find fun ways to practice letters and sounds (such as making objects out of letters, like a tree out of the letter T, a snake out of the letter S, etc.), and watch an occasional educational video together, such as *Sesame Street*'s "Getting Ready to Read."

And for you (last but not least!), we recommend formal assessment and follow-up intervention if necessary given your concerns about having dyslexia. It is never too late to learn to read or to improve your level of literacy, so don't forget to help yourself, too.

Q: *Other than poor performance on these tests you have mentioned, is there anything else in my child's performance that the psychologist would be examining?*

A: Yes, the psychologist will also be assessing more subtle measures of reading and language ability. These include:

- *Problems with verbal short-term memory.* As verbal short-term memory is sometimes affected by dyslexia, poor performance on subtests such as the WISC-IV Digit Span and other memory tests is often seen.
- *Word finding difficulties and verbal formulation problems.* Child-

ren with dyslexia sometimes have difficulty "coming up with the right word." As a result, they may be unusually quiet. They may also have relatively poor performance on tests such as the Boston Naming Test and the Expressive Vocabulary Test, tests that require the children to name pictures of objects or actions (i.e., "come up with" the right word for something).

- *Reversal errors.* Reversal errors include substituting similar letters, such as *b* and *d*. At one time reversal errors were considered the classic symptom of dyslexia. This has been found to be untrue, as there are many children with dyslexia who do not reverse letters and many children without dyslexia who do. However, the examiner will note if they do occur, because the presence of reversal errors in children over the age of nine is of important diagnostic significance. Normal readers of that age or older almost never make reversal errors. It is interesting to note that the reason for these errors has little to do with the visual system: *b* and *d* have similar sounds.

- *Lexicalizations.* This is a complicated word that has a simple definition. Lexicalizations involve substituting a real word when one is asked to read a nonreal word. For example, on the Word Attack subtest of the Woodcock–Johnson, a child is asked to read the word *bim*. Because this is an unfamiliar nonword, the child may make a real-word guess and identify the word as *boy*. Rather than try to sound out the word phonetically (because phonetic skills are weak), the child substitutes a whole-word guess that looks somewhat similar to the nonword.

- *Visual errors.* Visual errors occur when a child is presented with the word *bat* but reads it as *boat*. Instead of using phonics to sound out the word, she substitutes a word that is visually similar.

- *Dysfluency.* Children with dyslexia often demonstrate slow and labored reading. Their oral reading often includes such errors as substituting and omitting words.

- *Spelling errors.* It is very common for children with dyslexia to make *dysphonetic errors* on their spelling tests. Such errors include the omission, substitution, or inappropriate addition of a phoneme. These errors can include writing *expnen* for *explain, necrer* for *nature, eog* for *edge,* or *anmaganary* for *imaginary.*

Q: Even though my son is very bright, he was diagnosed with dyslexia. How can that be?

A: One of the benefits of performing intelligence testing as part of a thorough evaluation for dyslexia and other learning disabilities is that the professional or parent can frequently reassure the child with the information that he or she is indeed smart. By "smart" we mean that the child is at least of average intelligence and is able to learn grade-level concepts and skills. It is true that many children with learning disabilities, including dyslexia, are exceptionally bright, scoring in the above-average or superior range on intelligence testing. The list of well-known people with dyslexia is filled with individuals widely accepted as genius or brilliant; these include Albert Einstein, Pablo Picasso, and Leonardo da Vinci.

The fact that many people with dyslexia have excelled in creative pursuits such as painting, inventing, and creative writing seems to be due to more than coincidence. That is, it seems that it is fairly common for people with dyslexia to be highly talented in creative thinking and expression. We suggest allowing your son to try out his skills in a variety of creative fields such as art, music, drama, carpentry, and creative writing.

Although we recognize that having your child diagnosed with a learning disability may cause you to worry about his future, we remind you that there have been may advances in understanding and treating dyslexia. For your child to begin accepting that he has a learning disability, it will be important for you to do so as well.

The Testing's Completed: Now What Do I Do?

Once parents receive a diagnosis and report of the results, they often realize that the testing process was not an end in and of itself but only the beginning. A good evaluation should provide you with specific treatment recommendations that are tailored to your child's unique abilities. That said, we want to at least give you an idea of the more commonly recommended treatment strategies for dyslexia, as well as how you might explain this diagnosis to your child.

What Should I Tell My Child about the Diagnosis?

Although some parents worry that "labeling" their child's problems will somehow damage them or make them feel bad about themselves, the fact is that the majority of people (kids and grownups alike) find considerable relief in knowing that what they have been struggling with or suffering from actually has a name. By telling your child, in age-appropriate language, about dyslexia, you are validating what she has likely known for a long time—that she learns to read differently than most other kids and that she has yet to be taught in the right way. Telling her that everyone has strengths and weaknesses, or naming things your child is really good at and things that are harder for her, is also helpful in framing her reading difficulties for her. Use the results of the testing to describe her areas of strength. Point out all of her talents and interests, which will reassure her that, indeed, there are many things she can do well. Often children with dyslexia will show strengths in creative thinking and hands-on skills. If she is old enough, you might want to explain that the way her brain is wired makes it more difficult for her to hear the little sounds that make up words. Because of this, learning to read and spell has been harder for her. You will want to reassure her that this does not mean her brain or mind does not work well in general; she is as smart as her classmates (often smarter!) but just has difficulty in this one area. Citing some of the well-known successful people with dyslexia may also be helpful to her in accepting the diagnosis and to see that it does not mean she can't do well in any area that interests her. Leonardo da Vinci, writer Roald Dahl, actor Tom Cruise, athlete Dan O'Brien, and Albert Einstein are just a few of the many individuals with dyslexia who have pursued their dreams and found success.

Several books are now available for children and teenagers who have been diagnosed with learning disabilities. Because it is very common for children with dyslexia or any other learning disability to suffer from low self-esteem, it will be critical for you to help your daughter understand and accept her difficulties while promoting her strengths and interests. The school psychologist or guidance counselor may be a helpful resource should your daughter have trouble dealing with her academic struggles despite your support.

Q: As if my son's dyslexia weren't enough, now his teacher tells me he is having a lot of trouble following directions and staying organized at school. Why could that be, and is it related to his dyslexia? Does this mean I need to have him retested?

A: We often hear that a child with dyslexia has difficulties similar to your son's. Because many children with dyslexia have difficulty with general auditory processing, they often have trouble taking in spoken information at the rate at which most kids can. In addition to listening more slowly, affected kids may perceive information they hear out of sequence and/or inaccurately. They may have trouble tuning out background noise to hear what is being said to them. As a result, tasks such as following spoken directions become quite difficult.

Because problems with auditory processing interfere with a child's ability to take in spoken information, it may appear that an affected child is not paying attention to what is being said. Your son's teacher or you may have even wondered if he has attention-deficit/hyperactivity disorder (ADHD), inattentive type, because of his problems following directions or perhaps keeping up with a story someone is telling. Although it is important to note that the risk of a child with dyslexia also having ADHD is significantly higher than for a child who has no learning disability, many dyslexic children are misdiagnosed with ADHD because of auditory processing difficulties. (For more information on the indications of ADHD, see Chapter Seven, "Attention-Deficit/Hyperactivity Disorder.") If you suspect that your son truly has auditory processing problems rather than ADHD, we recommend an evaluation by a speech and language therapist or by a pediatric audiologist, who will perform a central auditory processing (CAP) evaluation. The latter exam tends to be quite expensive, however, and is not always covered by health insurance.

The observation that your child also has organizational problems is a common concern reported for students with dyslexia. Although the exact reason is not clear, it may be that, because the affected part of the brain in people with dyslexia is also involved in sequencing and the sense of time, their ability to plan and organize may be negatively affected as well. However, organizational difficulties are also a primary concern in people with ADHD, and so we recommend that you have your child evaluated for ADHD with the appropriate professional and methods (see Chapter Seven). If your son completed the dyslexia evaluation in the past year or so, recontact the evaluator and ask if he could either do a brief evaluation for ADHD or reexamine the test results to see if a diagnosis of ADHD is warranted. Talk to him about the teacher's concerns and ask him how he would recommend evaluating them. If it has been more than two years since your child received a complete evaluation, ask the evaluator whether a new evaluation or a referral to an additional professional (e.g., speech and language therapist) is warranted.

Treatment

Currently, it is widely accepted that the optimal teaching approach for students of all ages diagnosed with dyslexia is the use of one of the multisensory, sequential, phonics-based reading methods such as the Orton–Gillingham, Lindamood–Bell, or Wilson method. Although there is some variation among the different programs in exactly how they go about teaching phonemic awareness and enhancing phonological processing, the important common factor is the multisensory approach.

For example, children with dyslexia who receive the Orton–Gillingham approach, which has been shown to be one of the most effective methods for treating dyslexia, will first work on learning the letters and the sounds they represent. The child will do this visually (by seeing the written letter and by watching their mouths in the mirror as they say the letter), auditorily (by listening to the sound the letter makes), kinesthetically (by paying attention to the position and shape of the mouth when they say the letter, noticing how their mouth feels when they pronounce the letter or how their hands feel when they write the letter), and tactilely (by tracing the letter in sand or shaving cream). The program then builds from there, as the students learn to decode, comprehend, and write using a phonologically based, sequential method that incorporates other senses to enhance the learning process. It is success based in that every lesson ensures that the student will experience success; this is especially important because the typical person with dyslexia has usually had more than his fair share of failure and discouragement when it comes to reading.

Once it's determined that your child has dyslexia, you should request that she receive special education services for reading and related skills, such as spelling and writing. Given what we know about the importance of using a multisensory approach for students with dyslexia, you should insist that he receive instruction in one of these approaches. If the school offers you a program that you haven't heard of, ask for information about it to determine if it is multisensory and phonetically based. If your school system does not have a certified specialist available in any of the recommended multisensory methods, you will need to advocate for your child to obtain these services. This may involve locating an available specialist, either privately or in a neighboring school system, and holding the school responsible for covering the costs of servicing your son outside the system. Many parents find they need the assistance of an educational advocate to help them in the process of obtaining the necessary services for their children, but hopefully you will not need to take this step, given that it usually means that the school is not cooperating as you would like and involves out-of-pocket expenses for you.

The intensity of the multisensory services is very important. In general, it is recommended that a student receive at least three sessions, of forty-five to sixty minutes each, per week of a multisensory reading method. Most of these programs work best individually but usually can be provided to students in small groups if needed.

Q: My son was found to have dyslexia when he was in third grade, but now he is about to go off to college next year. Should we have him reevaluated to help determine what accommodations or treatment is appropriate for him at this time?

A: A reevaluation is often appropriate when the student with dyslexia is approaching college. Assuming that your son has received the appropriate intervention for dyslexia since about the third grade, when the problem was first diagnosed, he has likely improved significantly in his word decoding skills, spelling, reading comprehension, and writing skills. Although some students with dyslexia eventually decode and comprehend on grade level after receiving the proper instruction, it is common for people with dyslexia to continue to struggle with new or less familiar words. In addition, they tend to read and therefore comprehend written information at a slower rate than readers who do not have this problem. Because of this, your son may need to apply for the accommodation of extra time on exams, including entrance exams such as the SATs. To apply for extra time, he will need to have an evaluation that was completed in the preceding two years. Because the guidelines for extended time on the SATs and other tests like them are subject to change, you'll want to check that the evaluator is familiar with the type of information or evaluation the testing service needs to determine whether your child will qualify for extended time. Testing can also indicate whether your son may benefit from advance notice of large reading assignments to provide him with the extra time he will likely need.

Another accommodation that's often helpful to students with dyslexia is spelling assistance, such as with a spell-check device, or a provision that spelling errors will not count against the overall grade of the paper or test. Although this may seem to be giving unfair advantage to the student with dyslexia, it is common for people with dyslexia to continue to have relatively poor spelling skills even when they are capable of reading at age or grade level. This concern is rooted in the phonological processing problems that underlie dyslexia, which seem to make spelling a particularly difficult task. The evaluation can determine whether this is still a necessary accommodation for your son.

Because many students with dyslexia often have organizational difficulties, your son may benefit from maintaining a schedule of activities, assignment due dates, and other pertinent information. Testing may indicate whether he would benefit from formal organizational or study-skills tutoring. Some colleges will provide this service, or you may need to find a private tutor in the area for him.

Most colleges today will provide accommodations such as those described here with documentation of the student's disability within about two years of applying to college. It will be important to ask the college admissions office or office of student affairs of each of the schools he is interested in if they will provide the accommodations you are hoping to receive for him. If you have not had your son reevaluated recently, this should be completed prior to taking the SATs (if you are going to request extra time and certainly before he begins college).

Resources

Books for Parents

Adelizzi, J. U. (2001). *Parenting children with learning disabilities.* Westport, CT: Bergin & Garvey Press.

Clark, D. B., & Uhry, J. K. (1995). *Dyslexia: Theory and practice of remedial instruction.* Timonium, MD: York Press.—Describes dyslexia and the various methods of treating dyslexia, such as Orton–Gillingham. A classic, comprehensive book.

Shaywitz, S. (2003). *Overcoming dyslexia: A new and complete science-based program for reading problems at any level.* New York: Knopf.

Spafford, C. S., & Grosser, G. S. (1995). *Dyslexia: Research and resource guide.* Boston: Allyn & Bacon.

Organizations/Web Sites

International Dyslexia Association
www.interdys.org

Learning Disabilities Association of America
www.ldanatl.org

LD Online
www.LD.org

Things to Keep in Mind after You Receive the Report

If the evaluation was completed through the school system read the report and write down your questions, schedule and attend the team meeting, and bring up any questions you might have jotted down. *There are no dumb questions.* Professionals (ourselves included!) often talk over parents' heads and use terms that nonprofessionals don't know. Ask them to define their terms, and don't be satisfied until you really understand what they're talking about. If you have questions that aren't answered at the team meeting, schedule an appointment with the school psychologist.

If the evaluation was done independently. make sure you talk to the evaluator after receiving the report if you have any questions. Many evaluators will give you a heads-up on what to expect from the report, but *don't be afraid to ask questions.* We can't stress this enough. There is no way that any psychologist can anticipate every question. (Indeed, that was one of our primary incentives for writing this book.) Therefore, it's up to you to let them know what you need help understanding. You may also want to schedule a meeting with the school to go over the results and determine how best to integrate the recommendations into your child's school programming.

If your child was *evaluated both by the school and independently,* you may find yourself with two opposing viewpoints as to what treatment is most effective. Keep in mind what you want—namely, for your child to receive the correct services. Although you are your child's best advocate, if the school is reluctant to provide treatment even though the independent evaluation makes a strong case for treatment, you may need to engage the services of a professional advocate. (See Chapter Two for more information on how to go about doing that.)

Seven

Attention-Deficit/ Hyperactivity Disorder

Attention-deficit/hyperactivity disorder (ADHD) is a common disorder of childhood that affects 3 to 5 percent of school-age children. ADHD is a syndrome defined by the characteristic behaviors of inattention, impulsivity, and hyperactivity. Some children have primarily impulsive/hyperactive symptoms, others have primarily inattentive symptoms, and many children have a combination of inattentive and impulsive/hyperactive symptoms. To receive a diagnosis of ADHD, the child's symptoms must cause a significant amount of impairment in at least two different settings, such as home and school or work. ADHD is more prevalent in boys than in girls, and, by definition, the symptoms of the disorder must be present early in life (before the age of seven years). Although a fair number of children outgrow their symptoms of ADHD, approximately half of those diagnosed will continue to show symptoms into adulthood. As children grow into adolescence and adulthood, many of the hyperactive symptoms will subside, though the inattentive symptoms remain. We don't know what causes ADHD, but there is very strong evidence for an inherited component, as well as some known environmental risk factors, such as fetal alcohol syndrome, lead poisoning, and head trauma, that are associated with an increased risk for ADHD.

Psychological testing is not necessary to diagnose ADHD, because ADHD is considered a behavioral disorder. That is, the diagnostic criteria for ADHD are all focused on behavior, and any child who exhibits those behaviors according to the parameters set forth in the criteria can be diagnosed with ADHD. There is, however, a role for testing in diagnosing ADHD, and therefore psychological testing is very often

Q: My child is the opposite of hyperactive–it takes a tornado to get her moving–yet the psychiatrist diagnosed her with attention-deficit/hyperactivity disorder. How can this be?

A: It sounds as though your daughter has the inattentive subtype of ADHD. You're certainly not the only parent who has been confused by the use of the word *hyperactive* in the diagnosis of a child who isn't remotely hyperactive. Keep in mind that there are three subtypes of ADHD: predominantly hyperactive–impulsive type, predominantly inattentive type, and combined type.

---

part of an ADHD evaluation. When ADHD is diagnosed on the basis of an office visit with a doctor or on behavioral checklists alone, children who have disorders such as dyslexia, a nonverbal learning disability, depression, or anxiety may be misdiagnosed. Testing can also identify learning disabilities that sometimes co-occur with ADHD. Neuropsychological testing can also provide evidence that can help confirm the diagnosis of ADHD, particularly by evaluating a child's *executive functions*, discussed later in this chapter, which are sometimes weak in children with ADHD. Assessing these areas can help confirm a diagnosis of ADHD when your child's doctor is unsure and can also provide important information about a child's areas of weakness that can help the doctor devise the best treatment interventions.

You may know a child like Zach, the hyperactive, inattentive first grader whose teacher referred him for further evaluation. Zach had demonstrated problems with hyperactivity since preschool, and now, in first grade, it was nearly impossible for him to stay in his seat. Zach's pediatrician had originally told his parents not to worry because many of the behaviors Zach was exhibiting, such as excessive energy and difficulty sitting still for long periods of time, are part of normal behavior in preschoolers. However, when Zach's teacher requested that his parents look further at his difficulties, they took Zach back to his pediatrician, who then suspected ADHD and suggested a comprehensive evaluation.

Zach's evaluation was covered by insurance, so his pediatrician suggested that his parents seek an independent evaluation by a neuropsychologist. The psychologist began the evaluation by asking Zach's parents questions about his developmental history. They described Zach as a "colicky baby who rarely slept." As a toddler, he was always on the go and seemed to have no fears. He'd climb to the top of the play structure at the playground and jump down. They'd made frequent trips to the emergency room. They summed up Zach's early years by saying "He wore us out. Each day was a new challenge, and although we loved him dearly, he exhausted us with his constant need for our attention and his constant movement." Zach's preschool and kindergarten teachers also noted in his year-end evaluation that, although he was a delightful child, he had numerous difficulties completing his work and "keeping his hands to himself" and was always "talking out of turn."

After obtaining a thorough developmental history, the neuropsychologist completed a comprehensive evaluation of Zach. Throughout the testing process Zach was extremely talkative, fidgety, inattentive, and impulsive. He was, however, able to control his behavior when the examiner provided him with additional structure. Tests of cognitive ability and academic achievement indicated that Zach had an average IQ and was progressing well in all subjects, with the exception of writing tasks. He did, however, perform poorly on a number of tests of *executive functions*, including tests of auditory memory, visual organization, and attention. More important, behavior rating scales and checklists completed by Zach's parents and teachers indicated clinically significant symptoms of inattention, impulsivity, and hyperactivity. Taken together, Zach's history, performance on a number of tests of attention, and behavioral ratings indicated that he met the criteria for ADHD, Combined Type.

The neuropsychologist who evaluated Zach suggested that Zach and his parents talk to their pediatrician or a child psychiatrist about beginning a trial course of medication for Zach's symptoms. She also suggested that Zach receive school resource-room help with organization and study skills, along with a number of classroom accommodations, such as tasks broken into smaller components, preferential seating, frequent breaks, frequent feedback, and additional structuring of his day. Finally, she recommended that Zach's handwriting difficulties be evaluated more thoroughly by an occupational therapist. With these suggestions implemented, Zach's behavior improved considerably in the classroom and at home.

Diagnosing ADHD

ADHD evaluations can take a couple of different forms. Sometimes pediatricians or psychiatrists will complete an evaluation by asking you and your child questions about the frequency of different behaviors. Other times they will refer children for additional testing for the purposes described earlier.

What the Testing Evaluation Should Include:

A comprehensive evaluation for ADHD would include:

- An interview with the parent and child that includes information about the child's early development and family history for symptoms of ADHD
- Behavior rating scales, such as the CBCL, BASC, Conners' Rating Scales, and/or ADHD Rating Scale (the latter two are described later)
- Tests of cognitive ability and academic achievement (to rule out possible learning disabilities)
- Neuropsychological tests, including tests of executive functions

Tests of Executive Functions

To understand what these tests are measuring, it might be useful to think of executive functions as similar to the job that executive secretaries perform. They keep their boss's calendar, handle and prioritize their boss's correspondence, determine which phone calls are necessary for the boss to take, and organize most aspects of the day-to-day running of an office. A good executive secretary has to be able to think about many things simultaneously and decide which of those things are most important and which of them can wait. The frontal lobes of the brain do much the same thing for us. This area of the brain is responsible for planning, future-oriented behavior, attention, and self-regulation. Brain imaging research has confirmed what neuropsychological tests have indicated, that this part of the brain is different in people with ADHD. Although not all of those with ADHD perform poorly on tests of executive functions, many do, and the greater the number of impaired scores on executive function measures, the greater the likelihood that ADHD is present.

> **Executive functions** is a general term that refers to processes such as planning; organizational skills; the ability to focus one's attention, as well as the ability to know *where* to focus one's attention and the ability to maintain attention; and the ability to inhibit one's behavior.

Some of the more commonly used tests of executive functions include the following, which were described in detail in Chapter Four:

- California Test of Verbal Learning (CVLT) or Children's Auditory Verbal Learning Test (CAVLT)
- Stroop Color and Word Test
- Rey–Osterrieth Complex Figure
- Wisconsin Card Sorting Test
- Trails A and B
- Continuous Performance Test (CPT)
- Various tests of auditory and visual memory, such as those found on the Children's Memory Scale or the Wide Range Assessment of Memory and Learning

Additional tests include:

- *Freedom from Distractibility Index* from the WISC-III or *Working Memory Index* from the WISC-IV. This index is an indication of a child's ability to sustain attention, concentrate, and exert mental control. Mental control is the ability to listen to information (for example, an oral arithmetic problem such as "If Bobby has seven apples and John has three, how many apples are there altogether?") and then hold it in short-term memory while performing the operation.
- *Controlled Oral Word Association Test.* On this test the child is asked to rapidly generate a list of words beginning with each of three letters and/or to generate a list of words in a particular category. The test is scored by comparing the total number of words with the mean for children the same age. Qualitative observations can also be made, such as whether the child lost task set (forgot what he was supposed to be doing), generated perseverative responses (kept saying the same responses over and over), or "lost steam" (gave fewer responses as time progressed, which is an indication of loss of attention).

Behavior Rating Scales

Scales of behavioral functioning are a very important part of the evaluation process. Some of the more commonly used tests of behavioral functioning include the following, which were described in detail in Chapter Four:

- Child Behavior Checklist (CBCL)
- Behavior Assessment System for Children (BASC)

Other behavioral rating scales commonly used in ADHD evaluations include:

- *ADD-H Comprehensive Teacher's Rating Scale (ACTeRS)*, a behavior rating scale of a child's difficulties with attention, hyperactivity, social skills, and oppositionality in the classroom setting.
- *ADHD Rating Scale*, a measure that asks parents to rate the frequency of ADHD behaviors.
- *Parent SNAP (Swanson, Nolan, & Pelham) Checklist,* which assesses symptoms of inattentiveness, impulsivity, peer interactions, and hyperactivity.
- *Behavior Rating Inventory of Executive Functioning (BRIEF)*, a parent and teacher rating form of executive functions that measures behaviors such as the inability to inhibit (e.g., the child acts wilder or sillier than others in groups, interrupts others, gets out of her seat at the wrong time), the inability to organize materials (the child leaves the playroom a mess or keeps her room messy), the inability to shift cognitive set (the child gets stuck on one topic or activity or, after having a problem, stays disappointed for a long time), lack of emotional control (the child's mood changes frequently or he reacts more strongly to situations than other children do), and weakness in working memory (the child has a short attention span, is easily distracted by noises, activities, sights, etc., and needs help from an adult to stay on task).
- *Conners' Rating Scales*, measures of symptoms of ADHD. Includes parent and teacher rating forms.

Preparing for an ADHD Evaluation

If you are scheduled for the simpler type of evaluation for ADHD, you can prepare your child by telling her you're meeting with a doctor who will be asking her—and you—many questions. This type of evaluation is fairly brief, so you should be able to assure your child that you'll be all finished and on your way home within an hour. Most often this type of evaluation will be completed in a pediatrician's or psychiatrist's office. The doctor may spend much of the time talking alone with the parents, and thus your child may be uncomfortable or anxious sitting in the

Q: *The neuropsychologist who examined my son, Tyler, said he was an "absolute angel" during the testing, and as a result she saw few symptoms of inattention, hyperactivity, or impulsivity while testing him. Yet she diagnosed him with ADHD. How can you diagnose a child with ADHD when you didn't even see the symptoms?*

A: Believe it or not, it is not that unusual for us to see few ADHD symptoms in our office. Children with ADHD often perform at their best in new surroundings with novel challenges to keep them interested. They also perform best in structured settings. The evaluation process offers both of these, and, in addition, children benefit from the increased one-on-one attention they get. In this case the examiner must rely on the child's history, on behavior rating scales, and on interviews with parents and teachers. Sometimes the evaluator may decide to make a classroom visit so she can observe the behaviors firsthand, although that is not necessary to make the diagnosis. Conversely, problem behaviors that we *do* see during testing give us important evidence regarding the diagnosis. In other words, if a child has difficulty focusing in a novel, highly structured, one-on-one setting, then it is very likely that he would have much difficulty in less structured settings, such as home or a busy classroom.

Q: *So what types of behaviors do you typically see during testing?*

A: Behaviors that we commonly observe are fidgeting, frequent complaints about the length of testing ("When are we going to be done?" "Is this ever going to be over?" "Do we have to do that whole book?"), impulsive responses to tasks, requests for frequent breaks, difficulty shifting set (moving from one task to another), and poor attention in a variety of tasks. We often see hyperactivity, with kids commonly having difficulty staying in their seats. Children with ADHD will frequently make careless errors because they aren't paying sufficient attention to the task. For example, a child's performance on a written math test may be affected by lack of attention to the operational sign (e.g., adding the numbers instead of subtracting) or by not lining the columns up correctly on a long division problem.

Q: *The neuropsychologist who evaluated my child said he had ADHD and dyslexia. How does she know he has both? Couldn't an inability to concentrate and focus lead to poor ability to read?*

A: The neuropsychologist who evaluated your child likely noticed that your child had significant difficulties with phonological processing, the ability to perceive the distinct sounds that make up a word (see Chapter Six for more details on this ability). Although we sometimes see decreased performance on tests of academic achievement (including reading) in children with ADHD, it is not typical to see deficits in phonological processing. More typically, if a child with ADHD has problems with reading, they will show in the area of reading comprehension, quite possibly because of the attentional component that is necessary to effectively comprehend what they've read. Keep in mind that ADHD frequently occurs with dyslexia. In fact, ADHD occurs more frequently in people with dyslexia than it does in the population at large. In your child's case, it is important to treat both disorders, because treatments for the two disorders are different. For more information about treatments for dyslexia, see Chapter Six.

---

waiting room, wondering what everyone is saying about him. Let your child know that he may possibly be waiting for quite some time in the waiting room. You might want to have him bring something to do, like a Game Boy or book, so he doesn't get bored.

A more comprehensive evaluation, which includes testing, usually takes three to five hours to complete. You can help your child prepare for the evaluation by telling him that he'll be meeting with a doctor who will be asking him to do things such as solve problems, complete puzzles, answer questions, read, and write.

If your child is extremely hyperactive, you might be wondering how he'll be able to complete an evaluation in which he's supposed to sit still for long periods of time. Although it can be difficult for some kids, as we said earlier, most will benefit from the one-on-one attention and the increased structure of the testing situation. The key is to pick an evaluator who has experience assessing children with ADHD. However, even the best psychologists can have trouble, particularly if your child had a poor night's sleep the night before, didn't eat breakfast, or is angry about something that happened on the way to the psychologist's office. Therefore, it's important to make sure your child is well rested and well fed the day before the evaluation. Also try to limit stressful situations during the day before the evaluation. On the day of the evaluation, pack your child's favorite snacks or drinks to take along, and let him know that you'll do something special as soon as he's done, such as buying him a new Game Boy game on the way home or stopping at McDonald's for lunch. This is a permissible form of bribery that can help keep an unfocused child more focused.

Finally, if your child is already on medication before completing a comprehensive test battery, you'll want to find out from the evaluator whether your child should be on medication the day of testing. We generally recommend that children take their prescribed medications so that we can see how they perform at their best. This also gives us information about whether the medication is working. There are other times, however, when it might be useful to see children off medication, such as if there is a question about whether the child actually has ADHD or when there is a concern that the child no longer needs medication. We've even had children come to see us twice, once on medication and once off. This is likely to be necessary only when there is a question as to whether the medication is effective. Your child is unique, and there is no way to predict what will be called for in her case; just be sure to ask the evaluator ahead of time.

The Testing's Completed: Now What Do I Do?

As you saw in Chapter Five, all testing evaluation reports should conclude with a summary and recommendations for solving any problems identified by the tests. If the testing evaluation was done to clarify certain aspects of your child's diagnosis or to identify the best possible interventions for the child, your son or daughter might already be taking medication prescribed for ADHD. If not, the report may very well recommend such treatment. The evaluator's recommendations might also include accommodations via a Section 504 Plan or special education under the auspices of IDEA, both described in detail in Chapter Two.

Treatment

The best approach to treating ADHD appears to include a combination of stimulant medication and behavioral treatment in the home and/or school. The use of medication in children with ADHD has been studied

Q: My son was just diagnosed with ADHD by a psychologist, and I took his report to the school in the hope of getting services for him. The school told me that ADHD does not entitle my son to any special services. Is that true?

A: Children with ADHD are covered under the "Other Health Impaired" category of the Individuals with Disabilities Education Act (IDEA), and they are eligible for mandated special education services and accommodations *if they need them.* In other words, receiving a formal diagnosis of ADHD doesn't automatically entitle a child to services. To be eligible, the ADHD condition must have an adverse effect on his educational performance. If you feel the school is in error, you can talk to an educational advocate who can help you seek services for your child. You may also want to join an organization such as Children and Adults with ADHD (CHADD), which can provide you with up-to-date information regarding education and legal rights.

What Should I Tell My Child about the Diagnosis?

There is much material to help you with this question, and the resource list at the end of this chapter can get you started. Because there are a lot of misperceptions about ADHD, you'll want to start by educating your child about what the diagnosis is. Depending on the age of your child, the information can be as simple as "it's sometimes hard for you to concentrate, especially in school, so Dr. XX is going to give you medicine that will help you concentrate." If your child is first diagnosed in middle or high school, she probably already has an opinion about what ADHD is. You'll want to ask her about what she thinks it is and how she feels about it. You'll also want to make sure she has accurate information about the disorder and give her the right information as needed.

The psychologist who completed the testing and/or the prescribing physician can play an important role in this process. Ask them to meet with your child to talk about what ADHD is and how it can affect one's performance. This meeting does not need to be lengthy. In addition, you may want to check out some books at the library that can provide your child with age-appropriate information. Finally, if someone in your family also has ADHD (and it's likely someone does), have him talk to your child about what his experience has been.

very extensively, and if you could choose only one treatment for your child, research has shown that properly prescribed stimulants have the greatest effect. The most commonly used drugs are stimulant medications, such as Ritalin (methylphenidate), Dexedrine (dextroamphetamine), and Cylert (magnesium pemoline). Stimulants should be effective immediately when prescribed properly. It may take some time to find the right one, but it's usually worth the effort. If stimulants are not successful, your doctor may prescribe an antidepressant or a combination of medications, such as an antidepressant and a stimulant. There is also a new nonstimulant medication, Strattera (atomoxetine), that has been shown in research studies to be effective in treating symptoms of ADHD. Your doctor may also prescribe more than one drug if your child has another psychiatric condition, such as an anxiety disorder or depression.

When we diagnose a child with ADHD, we generally recommend that the parents talk to their doctors about the pros and cons of medication. If the child's ADHD is mild, the parents may wisely choose to try some other behavioral interventions (described later) first. Those behavioral interventions may be enough to effectively manage the symptoms. However, when we see children with severe ADHD symptoms, we often *strongly* recommend that the parents discuss the possibility of medication with their doctor. Whether you decide to use medication depends on how severe and pervasive your child's difficulties are. You may decide that you can manage your child's symptoms quite well at home, but his attentional problems at school make it difficult for him to learn. In that case you may decide, with your child's physician, that your child may need the drug only on school days. However, you may have a child who is extremely hyperactive and always "getting in other people's faces" to the point that he has no friends. Your home life may be fraught with dinnertime disasters and family vacations that cause more stress than they alleviate because of your child's symptoms. In this case, you may decide that medication is important both in and out of school.

Quite appropriately, parents whom we see usually have a long list of questions about what might be involved in treating a child's ADHD with medication. Addressing them all is outside the scope of this book, and we strongly advise you to insist on satisfactory answers to your questions from your child's prescribing physician. You can also get lots of reliable information on medications from the resources listed at the end of this chapter. The following are, however, a few of the most pressing questions that we hear from parents.

Q: How often does my child have to take medication?

A: This depends on the type of medication prescribed. The effects of some medications last only four hours, whereas others last all day. There are many benefits to an all-day medication, one being the fact that your child won't have to go to the nurse's office at noon to take his medication. The decision regarding which medication should be given should be made in consultation with your doctor. New medications and new delivery systems of old medications are constantly being researched and marketed, so it's a good idea to work closely with your doctor to find the type of medication that works best.

Q: Are there side effects to the stimulant medications?

A: The most commonly reported side effects include difficulty sleeping and loss of appetite. Sleep problems can be treated by giving your child his medicine earlier in the day, reducing the dose, or changing from a long-acting to a shorter-acting medication. Loss of appetite can be treated by adding calorie-enhanced meals or giving children "drug holidays."

Q: I've heard that medicating your child can lead to later drug use. Is this true?

A: The answer, in a word, is no. Research studies have not documented that the use of stimulant medication causes later drug use. In fact, researchers such as Dr. Tim Wilens and Dr. Tom Spencer, our colleagues at Massachusetts General Hospital, studied the association of medication and later drug use. They expected to find no association between the two. What they found surprised them. When they looked at children who were treated with stimulant medication, they found *lower* rates of drug use during adolescence! Although we can only speculate on why this occurs, it may have something to do with the fact that children on stimulant medications are less impulsive and thus less likely to impulsively try illegal drugs. This finding is very important to consider when deciding whether to begin a medication trial with your child.

Although medication may be the treatment of choice for many children, you may want to try other methods before trying medication, or you may find that medication alone is not enough to completely treat your child's symptoms. Other treatments may include:

- Behavior therapy for the child and/or parents
- Preferential seating in the classroom to limit distractibility
- Increased structure and step-by-step reminders to help children organize their approaches to tasks
- "Chunking" longer tasks into smaller, more manageable segments
- Frequently repeating directions, preferably with direct eye contact
- Tutoring in study and organizational skills
- Testing in a separate room to limit distractions
- Giving permission to tape classroom lectures or providing access to notes from another student
- Tutoring in specific course content when needed
- Reducing the required number of courses per semester during college
- Holding more regular conferences with teachers to review progress
- Encouraging the use of homework assignment books for daily work and large calendars for long-range planning

It has been our experience that a combination of drug and behavioral treatments is most effective. Each child and family is individual, and what works for one family won't necessarily work for another. Finding the right treatment requires a collaboration among you, the evaluator, your child's teacher, and a medical doctor (pediatrician or child psychiatrist). For advice on making sure that you make optimal use of your child's test report and the evaluator's recommendations in arriving at treatment decisions, see the sidebar "Things to Keep in Mind after You Receive the Report" in Chapter Six.

Resources

There are literally hundreds of books, tapes, and Web sites available to parents and children who are interested in learning more about ADHD. Not all books are created equal, however, and some books have little basis in current research. Our best advice is to look for books that are written by qualified people who are affiliated with medical schools and/or colleges and universities. What we've presented here is just a short list of some of our favorite resources.

Books for Parents

Barkley, R. A. (2000). *Taking charge of ADHD: The complete, authoritative guide for parents* (rev. ed.). New York: Guilford Press.

Barkley, R. A., & Benton, C. (1998). *Your defiant child: Eight steps to better behavior.* New York: Guilford Press.

Dendy, C. Z. (1995). *Teenagers with ADD: A parents' guide.* Bethesda, MD: Woodbine House Books.—A great resource for helping parents cope with the ups and downs of raising a teen with ADHD.

Dendy, C. Z. (2000). *Teaching teens with ADD and ADHD: A reference guide for teachers and parents.* Bethesda, MD: Woodbine House Press.

Greene, R. (2001). *The explosive child: A new approach for understanding and parenting easily frustrated, chronically inflexible children.* New York: HarperCollins.—One of the best books for understanding and treating aggressive, noncompliant children. Although many children with ADHD won't fit into this category, the techniques presented in the book are very useful to parents of children with ADHD.

Hallowell, E., & Ratey, J. (1994). *Driven to distraction: Recognizing and coping with attention deficit disorder from childhood through adulthood.* New York: Pantheon Books.

Nadeau, K., Littman, E., & Quinn, P. (2000). *Understanding girls with AD/HD.* San Diego, CA: Advantage Books.

Wilens, T. (2001). *Straight talk about psychiatric medications for kids.* New York: Guilford Press.—The best book for parents on the subject of medication for kids. Includes detailed information on medications used to treat ADHD.

Books for Children

Nadeau, K., Dixon, E., & Rose, J. (1997). *Learning to slow down and pay attention: A book for kids about ADD.* Washington, DC: Magination.—A self-help book for kids ages nine to twelve.

Roberts, B. A. (1998 & 1999). *Phoebe's lost treasure* and *Phoebe's flower's adventures: That's what kids are for.* Silver Spring, MD: Advantage Books.—For children in grades 2 to 4.

Books for Teens

Nadeau, K., & Carter, S. (1998). *Help4ADD@high school.* San Diego, CA: Advantage Books.—Written for teens in a format that allows them to "surf" for information. Provides information about high school problems such as sex, dating, social life, family difficulties, and getting ready for college.

Videos

Barkley, R. A. (1993). *ADHD–What can we do?* New York: Guilford Press.

Organizations/Web Sites

Attention Deficit Disorder Association
www.add.org
—Provides current information about treatment, research, legal, and school issues as they relate to ADHD.

Children and Adults with Attention-Deficit/Hyperactivity Disorder (CHADD)
www.chadd.org
—One of the best Web sites, providing information on topics such as current research, legal issues, local support groups, and treatment.

Eight

Nonverbal Learning Disorders and Asperger Syndrome

Over the past few years, nonverbal learning disorders (NLD) and Asperger syndrome (AS) have been receiving a lot more attention in research, clinical settings, and the media. We think this is partly a product of a rather dramatic rise in incidence that can't be explained simply by the fact that parents and professionals are becoming better at picking up on these problems. To explain this increase, scientists are looking at the role of genes passed on by parents who may have some of the traits of the disorders, speculating that these genes may then somehow become more concentrated or exaggerated in the children. Researchers have also found some association between children with NLD or AS and other close relatives, such as an uncle or a grandparent, who have shown signs of the disorders. Studies of such associations have also revealed some link between a higher risk for NLD and AS in children and the incidence of autism, bipolar disorder, and schizophrenia in family members.

It is now estimated that about 1 percent of the population has NLD, which translates into about 2.7 million children and adults currently. The incidence of AS is estimated now to be about one out of every five hundred children in the United States, making AS a more commonly diagnosed problem than Down syndrome. Both AS and NLD occur more often in boys than girls, with AS affecting four boys for every girl (4:1 ratio).

Justin's parents had been concerned about his lack of friends ever since kindergarten. At their parent–teacher conference, Justin's third-grade teacher reported that he seemed to have difficulty knowing how to interact with other kids; in addition, he was now having trouble with schoolwork. Apparently, Justin wasn't always able to understand what he read, though he had learned to read early. He was also finding it hard to write very well, and his penmanship was often sloppy. At home his parents had noticed that his outbursts were becoming more frequent and that he often didn't get the jokes his siblings made. When his teacher said she suspected something called a "nonverbal learning disorder" and recommended that Justin have a team evaluation, they agreed and were glad to be taking steps to try to understand him better.

Sandra's mom remembers that when Sandra was very young one of the many professionals they consulted said that she may have something called "Asperger syndrome." Now, many years later, the psychologist who had just completed a neuropsychological evaluation with Sandra said the same thing. He explained that their concerns regarding her rather odd, flat way of speaking and almost obsessive interest in space were related to AS. After reading up on this disorder, Sandra's parents were amazed at how closely she resembled the children discussed in the books and found relief in knowing that help was available.

Professionals are almost sure that, although they are often talked about together, NLD and AS are not the same thing. But because children diagnosed with NLD and AS often share many characteristics and benefit from similar interventions, it is useful to speak about them in this way. Both of these diagnoses are considered neurobehavioral disorders, or brain-based problems that affect most aspects of functioning—behavior, learning, social skills, and emotional well-being. With this in mind, the label *nonverbal learning disorder* seems a bit of a misnomer, as it is not just a learning disability but one that affects almost all domains of the child's life. In addition, recent research and clinical experience have taught us that the deficits are not simply in the nonverbal realm. For example, many children with NLD have problems with abstract language and reading comprehension.

Because one of the primary weaknesses in both NLD and AS is information processing, some professionals have suggested renaming NLD *information processing disorder (IPD)*. Others have said it should be called a *neurointegrative disorder,* because affected children have trouble pulling together information usefully in order to adapt and learn as they should. Still others see the primary deficit as social skills and argue that NLD should be considered a so-called social disorder.

> **Information processing** refers to the way in which people take in information from the environment and how efficiently they use it to learn or respond.

AS has traditionally been thought of as part of the autism spectrum, and some children diagnosed with AS appear to have full-blown autism as toddlers or preschoolers but then advance in their communication and social skills beyond the typical autistic child's abilities. Others may never seem fully autistic but may share many of the core features, though less severely. Rather than appearing to be completely in his own world, for example, the child with AS may seem only mildly attuned to or interested in other people. Some then say that AS is simply "high-functioning autism" (HFA), meaning that people with AS have been only mildly affected by autism or have been able to compensate well for their deficits. Although this idea is under great debate, most of the main researchers and clinicians in the field agree that HFA and AS will emerge as distinct categories with more study. Though there may be overlap in the symptoms, it is important for practitioners to acknowledge the differences that exist by giving an accurate diagnosis (see Chapter Nine for more on HFA) so that the child's precise problems can be addressed appropriately in treatment.

Diagnosing Nonverbal Learning Disorder and Asperger Syndrome

The deficits seen in children with either NLD or AS fall into three broad areas, as already mentioned: information processing, social skills, and motor coordination and output. We think it's helpful to break these skills down further so that you can see how deficits in these three key areas basically affect all major aspects of the child's life.

Understanding the Deficits

Cognitive Skills

Although children with NLD and AS are typically quite verbal and often gifted in their language skills, we usually find a big gap between their verbal and nonverbal skills on intelligence testing. That is, on a test such as the WISC-IV, we would expect to see a significant difference (usually greater than 10 points) between the child's Verbal Comprehension score (higher) and Perceptual Reasoning score. Not all kids diagnosed with AS will show this profile, though, whereas it is virtually essential for a child diagnosed with NLD to demonstrate this big split in scores.

This finding alone signals a relative weakness in a group of skills governed mainly by visual–spatial and visual–motor processing, organization, and performance (e.g., drawing, writing, assembling things). It also suggests that the interplay or communication between various aspects of the brain is not working as effectively as it should. If it were, we would not find big pockets of weaknesses such as the major verbal–nonverbal gap. As a result of this breakdown in communication among brain functions, the child with NLD or AS has trouble pulling together information from the world in a consistently useful way; this then affects his ability to respond, adapt, and learn. The cognitive style of these children is often described as their having trouble "seeing the forest for the trees," the trees (details) being what they focus on rather than the forest (the full gestalt or "big picture"). Justin, for example, usually has trouble getting the point of movies or books because he gets so caught up in details. Cause-and-effect reasoning, too, has sometimes been found to be difficult for these kids, a finding that has implications for all types of learning.

Learning/Academics

Though kids like Justin with NLD or AS are usually strong readers in that they can decode words often above grade level, their ability to understand or summarize what they have read is typically impaired. This impairment is demonstrated on achievement or educational testing by a gap between the child's word reading skills score and reading comprehension score (much lower). One of the main reasons for this discrepancy is that children with AS and NLD tend to have trouble making inferences or getting the gist of what they hear and see; they prefer literal, black-and-white reasoning to abstract "gray" thinking. If the text they read is literal or factual in nature (e.g., "The cactus is a desert plant that is covered in sharp thorns"), they typically won't have a problem understanding it. But as soon as they are required to draw conclusions, make predictions, or "read between the lines" of the story, kids with NLD or AS often struggle. This type of reading comprehension is

Q: My son was tested through the school system, and they found that his nonverbal IQ score was almost thirty points lower than his verbal IQ score. He did poorly on reading comprehension and math, too. The school psychologist said he had a "specific learning disability" but didn't say anything about a nonverbal learning disorder, which is what I suspect from what I've been reading. How can I get more information about my child's learning style and functioning?

A: Because the school systems currently do not diagnose learning or behavioral disorders the way medical or mental health professionals tend to do, to some extent their hands are tied when it comes to identifying something like NLD. The school psychologist may suspect such a disorder for your child but may not label it as such. You need more testing to determine whether or not the diagnosis of NLD is appropriate and perhaps to rule out AS. We recommend that you obtain a neuropsychological evaluation with a psychologist who has a lot of experience with NLD and AS. Talk to the school system about this; if they support your decision to get a neuropsychological evaluation, they may help cover the cost should your insurance fail to do so.

By the way, we see many school systems still using a child's Full Scale IQ score as the best estimate of his intelligence even when there is a significant difference between the verbal and nonverbal IQ scores. As the Full Scale IQ score is essentially an average of the other scores (which are assumed to be within about ten points of each other), it has little or no meaning for children who have a major split between their verbal and nonverbal scores. We typically find that the higher score, in this case the verbal IQ score, reflects the child's intelligence potential and should be used in comparison with other test scores to figure out the child's true strengths and weaknesses. If the school system has used your child's Full Scale IQ score as an estimate of his potential/ability, its interpretation of what represents a strength and a weakness will be inaccurate and invalid.

---

usually part of the curriculum by third or fourth grade, so it is often then that this concern will arise. If ten-year-old Harry, who was diagnosed last year with NLD, read the sentence "Darkness passed over Sam's face as he realized Sara was lost forever," he would likely miss the emotional implication (sadness, grief) and understand "lost" literally (e.g., Sara could not be found as opposed to having died, etc.).

Written expression is a complex skill involving the ability to put ideas into writing in a legible, organized manner. Skills such as capitalization, grammar, and punctuation are also considered aspects of written expression.

Probably the biggest academic problem among children with AS and NLD, though, is *written expression*. Not only is the physical act of writing often difficult and slow, but also the multiple tasks required when writing a paper or answering an open-ended test question are frequently overwhelming. One needs to first come up with something to write about, organize the separate ideas while keeping in mind the overall topic of the paper, hold these ideas in working memory while physically transferring them from thought to writing, and so forth. Even brief writing assignments have been known to trigger some of the worst tantrums, or "meltdowns," for these kids, and parents are routinely frustrated by these reactions, especially given that their child is often so verbally bright.

Math skills are notoriously weak in children with NLD but may not be so for children with AS. These skills have traditionally been thought of as more nonverbal in nature, but there is often a lot of reading comprehension that goes along with math these days. Word problems, for example, require children to understand the information read, infer what operation (e.g., subtraction, addition) they need to perform, line the numbers up right on their paper, and then make the right calculation. Thus there are many opportunities for things to break down in doing math for a child with NLD or AS.

Like written expression, homework completion seems to be a universal problem for children with NLD or AS. Again, the multitasking involved in doing homework is enormous and requires effective organization—a known area of weakness for these kids. Children with NLD and AS often work quite slowly, and they become fatigued and frustrated easily as a result.

Language/Communication Skills

Though we've already emphasized the generally strong verbal skills in children diagnosed with NLD and AS, an important clarification needs to be made. Talking about fact-related information comes easily to these kids; children with AS in particular have been known to go on for excessive lengths of time about their preoccupations with dinosaurs, robotics, space, and other particular interests. However, when it comes

Asperger Syndrome and Nonverbal Learning Disorders: Similarities and Differences

Similarities	Differences
• Lower nonverbal IQ score (always for NLD; usually for AS) • Academic weaknesses in written expression, reading comprehension, and usually math • Fine-motor skill weaknesses • Gross-motor coordination weaknesses • Poor social skills, especially in reading social cues and making inferences • Problems with abstract language and pragmatics • Difficulty paying attention • Problems with organization • Trouble "shifting gears" • Information/sensory processing problems • Problems with emotional control, outbursts, withdrawal, anxiety	• Math skills may not be a serious weakness for children with AS but are almost always a concern for children with NLD • Drawing skills or interest in drawing may be strong for kids with AS but usually not so for kids with NLD • Social skill impairment is usually greater for children with AS • Some children with AS will speak in a monotone voice and have a stiff, rigid way of interacting—moreso than children with NLD • The sensory integration issues are usually greater for children with AS • Children with AS may have more intense preoccupations with specific areas of interest

to reading comprehension, kids with NLD and AS have trouble understanding the figurative nature of language, gestures, and other types of communication. Idioms such as "You're pulling my leg!" or "I'm kinda on the fence on this one" are often confusing to them, and a facial expression that shows fear followed by laughter makes no sense. Sarcasm and jokes may be hard for affected kids to get, but some have been known to have a pretty good sense of humor despite these weaknesses.

Social communication skills, called *pragmatics,* tend to be problematic for children with AS and NLD. Sustaining eye contact, responding to a greeting, starting a conversation, taking turns when talking or playing, and sharing interest in what another person is saying or doing tend to be relative weaknesses in these children.

> **Prosody** refers to the way a person stresses certain sounds and words when speaking. Children with AS will sometimes display a lack of prosody, giving their voices a monotone quality.
>
> **Pedantic speech**, also sometimes characteristic of people with AS, is an overly detailed, formal way of talking.

Kids diagnosed with AS, like Sandra, also sometimes have monotone voices, sometimes referred to as problems with *prosody. Pedantic speech* is also a fairly common feature of AS, which involves rather dull, encyclopedia-like verbalizations.

Social Skills

As you might guess, problems with pragmatics can cause a child with NLD or AS to stand out among his peers in a negative way. In addition to difficulty with things such as eye contact or keeping up with the natural give-and-take of conversation, affected kids often have problems reading social cues. This seems to be a result of many factors—problems getting the gist or subtle meanings of certain behaviors and comments, difficulty paying attention to what is going on, and trouble using past experience to understand what is happening in the present situation. Generalizing between one type of interaction or situation and the next is typically hard for children and adults with NLD or AS, and they tend to start fresh with every encounter. This contributes to the trouble we see in adapting or "going with the flow" of social interaction, and there is often a stilted, rigid quality to the way in which people with NLD or AS behave.

Another social concern that we think is a bit misunderstood is the tendency for kids with NLD or AS to be loners. Many people interpret this to mean that affected children are simply not interested in other people, that they just prefer to be alone. However, the majority of children we have worked with express a great longing for friendships and peer acceptance but are often anxious or unsure as to how to go about connecting with others. Older kids and adolescents may pull back from social interaction as a result of being rejected so often that they are wary of trying again.

The fact that most of the children with NLD or AS have gross-motor coordination problems often dissuades them from gravitating toward sports or other organized peer activities that are centered around physical activity. Given that these types of activities make up a lot of the social life of typical children and serve as opportunities for friendships and social interaction, this deficit puts them at yet another social disadvantage; they lose out on this otherwise common way to enhance self-esteem and end up feeling different and left out.

Motor Skills

The weaknesses in large-muscle coordination and strength typical of children with AS or NLD often make them appear clumsy and lead to great difficulty learning to do things such as riding a bicycle (if they can do so at all). Fine-motor skills may be relatively weak as well, particularly for children with NLD, who have associated handwriting and drawing difficulties. Here is sometimes another area that distinguishes NLD-diagnosed children from those with AS: kids with AS are sometimes very good at drawing and may become avid artists. The subject of their artwork, though, tends to take on a *perseverative* quality, in that they become stuck on a particular object or topic and repetitively draw it. Twelve-year-old Felicia, for example, loved to draw traffic lights—from all angles and in different settings, but always traffic lights. Fourteen-year-old Steven's pictures caused alarm for his parents, as he tended to draw violent, scary scenes over and over. A certain subset of kids may show a preoccupation with violence, which does not necessarily mean that they are prone to acting violently but that they may find this a way to express their anger or fears.

Perseverative behavior means that a person has trouble stopping a given act or transitioning to new activities or ways of thinking. Children who have perseverative tendencies often have trouble accepting change and "going with the flow."

Sensory Processing/Integration

Although this area alone warrants an entire book (and there are some good ones available, see the Resources at the end of this chapter), what we are talking about here is a tendency for kids with NLD and AS in particular to have a nervous-system-based problem with accurately perceiving, interpreting, and/or responding to sources of stimulation from the environment or inside their own bodies (e.g., emotional arousal or the sensation of having to go to the bathroom). We refer to these problems in perception usually as *hypersensitivity* (overly sensitive) or *hyposensitivity* (undersensitive).

A common area of hypersensitivity in children with NLD and AS is in the auditory realm, or a heightened sensitivity to sound. So, large group activities such as birthday parties, going to the mall, or eating in the school cafeteria may be overwhelming and quite stressful for these kids. This also tends to make affected kids easily distracted, as they may have trouble discriminating between unessential background noise and important information. When eight-year-old Pedro is in class, his neighbor's finger tapping seems as loud and as attention grabbing as his teacher's lecture; as a result, he misses a lot of what he is supposed to be learning in school.

Another sensory area in which many children with NLD and AS often experience problems is the tactile, or touch, system. Both an overreaction to touch (e.g., difficulty tolerating hair brushing, nail clipping, textured foods, certain clothing, or unexpected hugs or touches) and underreaction to pain may exist. The oversensitivity to touch may make some children resistant to playing with peers, as kids' interactions often include physical contact.

Kids with NLD and AS can also have sensory processing/integration problems that involve their awareness of their bodies in space, balance, and coordination. Difficulties with perceiving information from within their bodies makes regulating and understanding emotions hard for some kids, particularly because they may not be very good at sensing when they are becoming frustrated until it's too late and they blow up. Likewise, we have seen many children with sensory integration dysfunction have trouble with toilet-training because, as mentioned, they do not always register cues from their bodies that they have to "go" and accidents result.

Sensory integration dysfunction, or **SID**, is a medical diagnosis involving the nervous system. Children with SID have difficulty taking in or interpreting information from the environment or the body itself in an accurate and useful way. This then affects how they respond to stimuli—sometimes their response is too extreme and sometimes they underreact.

Executive Functions

Here is a fancy term for a group of skills that help us carry out the business of everyday life. For a more thorough explanation, see Chapter Seven on attention-deficit/hyperactivity disorder (ADHD), as this is the group of skills most affected by and related to ADHD. Briefly, these skills include paying attention, keeping impulses in check (censoring and filtering), sustaining effort, thinking and behaving flexibly, planning, and organizing. It may not be much of a stretch to claim that all kids with NLD and AS have at least some executive-function-based weaknesses, usually in sustained attention, flexible thinking, and organization.

What do these problems look like in real life? Well, affected kids will typically have trouble focusing in school or on homework, tend to have problems shifting gears in terms of their thinking or behavior, and find it hard to keep track of things or manage large assignments. Some parents wonder then whether their children with NLD or AS should also be diagnosed with ADHD, as they meet most if not all of the criteria. Technically, problems with executive functions are subsumed under the NLD or AS diagnosis, and a separate ADHD diagnosis is indicated only when the ADHD symptoms are more severe than what we would expect in a child with AS or NLD. Nevertheless, kids with NLD and AS often benefit from the interventions recommended for children with ADHD, including classroom accommodations and stimulant medication (see Chapter Seven).

Emotions/Behavior

Last, but certainly not least, NLD and AS tend to have an impact on children's emotional and behavioral functioning. As we've already explained, the underlying neurological problems affect learning and social skills in a number of ways. These problems also greatly affect how children feel, understand feelings within themselves and in others, and respond to an often confusing, overwhelming world.

Likely because of the difficulties they have with making sense of the world around them, it is very common for children diagnosed with AS or NLD to be quite anxious. If your child has AS or NLD, he may seem nervous and fearful, often avoiding situations that may prove stressful. This includes events that would typically seem fun for kids, such as birthday parties, fairs and carnivals, the mall, arcades, and organized peer group activities. Related to anxiety, we often hear about sleep difficulties, irritability, angry outbursts, and frequent meltdowns in children with NLD or AS.

Tantrums, or meltdowns, also tend to occur more frequently in these children due to problems with flexibility in thinking, sometimes referred to as difficulty with *shifting set* or perseveration. Shifting set is an executive-function-based skill that contributes to adaptability, or the capacity to shift from one idea or behavior to the next, depending on the context. So when Nathan's mom asks him to shut off the TV because it's time for dinner, he has significantly more trouble than the typical kid letting go of his current agenda ("I want to watch television") and shifting to a new one ("I need to go eat dinner now"). When kids are faced with more and more demands from their environment to shift from one thing to another, particularly at a rapid pace, the result is usually stress and anxiety. Too many demands will often lead to a major meltdown or total withdrawal from the child. At the very least, affected kids come across as oppositional, or stubborn, in that they have trouble complying with limits or demands for change placed on them.

We also see these kids preferring order and routine; when their safe, predictable schedule is interrupted or changed, again there is typically a surge of anxiety or stress. Aside from the fact that their trouble with adapting to change is working here, children and adults with NLD and AS seem to take comfort in knowing exactly what they can expect next; it is the unpredictable aspects of life that can be intolerable.

Another factor that contributes to behavioral concerns such as meltdowns or shutdowns (withdrawal) is the affected child's difficulty with self-monitoring and insight. *Self-monitoring* refers to the ability to tune in to oneself; here we mean the child's capacity to sense when he is becoming frustrated, anxious, or overwhelmed. Insight, or the ability to make connections between emotional states and the possible reasons for why they arise (a form of cause-and-effect reasoning), is typically quite limited in people with AS or NLD. As a result, it can be hard to get affected kids to understand the factors that contribute to their sadness or anxiety; without making these important links, it is difficult to make sense of one's experience and work to change it.

Related to limitations in insight, children with NLD and AS often have trouble accurately inferring how others might feel in certain situations and why. We have found that, though affected kids can often label the emotions implied by facial expressions ("He looks sad"), their skills may break down when they are asked why the person feels this way. Rather than assuming that this means that people with NLD or AS are not capable of *empathy*, we believe this repre-sents their difficulty with infer-ential reasoning and cause-and-

> **Empathy** is the ability to put ourselves in another person's place. By identifying with the other person, we understand how she is feeling and can respond ap-propriately—for example, consoling her after she has gotten hurt.

effect thinking, particularly when it comes to something as ambiguous as emotions. Feelings are an abstract concept, and, as we've discussed before, there is typically a strong, neurologically based preference for literal, black-and-white information in this population.

What the Testing Evaluation Should Include

Usually the type of evaluation that your child will need first will be a neuropsychological evaluation that looks at most or all of the areas dis-cussed here. For most kids, the testing will take about four to six hours, sometimes less. You can have your child tested through the public school system, but the school system will be able only to describe the

---

Q: My daughter was diagnosed with Asperger syndrome when she was about five years old. Now I'm wondering if she also has obsessive–compul-sive disorder (OCD) because the way she plays is so repetitive, she paces back and forth, and she can't seem to get her mind off certain ideas. She also does little things like putting all her books in a certain order. What do you think?

A: Although some children with AS will become so compulsive in their behavior and obsessional in their thinking that a separate diagno-sis of obsessive–compulsive disorder is warranted, for the most part what you've described tends to be par for the course with AS. Many af-fected kids will behave similarly to your daughter, and in fact these con-cerns are included in the *Diagnostic and Statistical Manual* (DSM-IV), which is the manual used by mental health professionals and many doc-tors to categorize and diagnose many types of disorders. Should these problems begin to interfere with her life, your daughter may benefit from some of the strategies proven useful for children with OCD, in-cluding cognitive–behavioral therapy and medication.

---

concerns, not diagnose the problem. It can be helpful to your child to receive a formal diagnosis of NLD or AS, because more and more school systems have specific classes and resources for affected kids. These kids are also more likely to need specialized placement, which you will probably want the public school system to pay for if your child cannot succeed in the public school setting. Having a formal diagnosis and solid documentation of your child's strengths and weaknesses can greatly help with this process.

A full neuropsychological evaluation is typically necessary for accurate and informed diagnosis of an NLD or AS. A full battery for NLD or AS should include:

- Intelligence testing
- Achievement/education testing
- Assessment of visual–spatial and visual–motor skills
- Language skills evaluation
- Assessment of executive functions
- Sensorimotor and neuromotor skills screen
- Social and behavioral assessment

Testing is often the deciding factor in distinguishing NLD from AS. Though the general profile is often similar as far as test results go, there are important subtleties that the evaluator should look for, including the severity of the social impairment (usually worse for kids with AS), math skills (usually worse in children with NLD), drawing/visual–motor integration skills (sometimes better in kids with AS), and factors such as prosody, pedantic speech, and degree of stiltedness in interaction (usually more prevalent among children with AS).

In addition to a thorough history of your child, the evaluation should consist of the following tests. Though the names of the measures may vary, the skills that they are designed to assess should be similar to those listed for each.

A Measure of Intelligence

As we've mentioned before, the results of the WISC-IV, DAS, or Stanford–Binet will likely indicate a significant difference between the child's verbal IQ and nonverbal IQ scores, the latter being lower. Again, although the majority of children diagnosed with AS will show this profile, it is not essential for the diagnosis. Conversely, it is fully expected for an NLD diagnosis.

Achievement/Educational Testing

A full battery of achievement testing should be administered, such as the WIAT-II or the Woodcock–Johnson. If not a battery, then individual measures of word decoding, reading comprehension, calculation skills, applied math and math reasoning, and written expression should be given. At least by about third to fourth grade, these results may show relative weaknesses in reading comprehension, math (more often for kids with NLD), and written expression.

Visual–Spatial/Visual–Motor Tests

Many different measures are available that examine these types of skills. Although we tend to use the Developmental Test of Visual Motor Integration (VMI), the Rey–Osterrieth Complex Figure Test, subtests of the WISC-IV or DAS, and sometimes the Hooper Visual Organization Test, you may see tests such

The **Test of Visual Perceptual Skills (TVPS)** is a measure of many different aspects of visual–spatial and visual–perceptual skills. It is made up of several subtests, including tests of visual memory, visual discrimination, visual closure, and form constancy.

as the Test of Visual Perceptual Skills (TVPS), Judgment of Line Orientation, or Bender Visual Motor Gestalt Test used. Usually weaknesses in these skills will be found, but some children with AS may have adequate drawing abilities. Visual organization concerns are almost always noted.

Language Tests

Though we tend to refer children for a full speech and language evaluation when we find concerns with figurative language, pragmatics, and other language-related skills, some psychologists may include tests such as the WIAT-II Oral Expression subtest when they suspect NLD or AS.

Executive-Function-Based Tests

Chapter Four provides a more extensive list and test descriptions, but you should find that at least tests of sustained attention, working memory, impulse control, flexibility and shifting set, and organization will be administered. These include measures such as the Wide Range Assessment of Memory and Learning (WRAML); Children's Memory Scale (CMS); California Verbal Learning Test for Children's Version; NEPSY, Wisconsin Card Sorting Test; Children's Category Test (a visual test of flexibility in problem solving similar to the Wisconsin Card Sorting Test); Trail Making Test, Trails A and B; Stroop Color and Word Test; Conners' Continuous Performance Test, and Rey–Osterrieth Complex Figure Test. Generally, we would expect to find relative weaknesses on many of these tests.

Sensorimotor/Neuromotor Tests

These tests examine sensory processing and motor functioning to determine if there are any differences between the left and right hands in terms of perception, output, and strength. Tests such as the Finger Tapping Test, Grooved Pegboard, Finger Agnosia, Fingertip Writing, Hand Dynamometer Grip Strength, and Lateral Dominance Exam may be used for this purpose.

Though not always, the findings on these tests will sometimes indicate that the child has right-hemisphere-based weakness. Because of

---

Sensorimotor/Neuromotor Tests

Dynamometer Grip Strength test. Looks at a person's hand strength in both the left and right hands; assesses whether or not there is a big difference between the left and right sides

Finger Agnosia Test and Fingertip Writing. Examines a person's ability to perceive stimulation accurately through touch

Finger Tapping Test. Tests for a person's ability to isolate and control the pointer finger of each hand, motor output speed, and right- and left-sided differences

Grooved Pegboard. A test of fine-motor control, manipulation skills, motor output speed, and right- and left-sided differences

Lateral Dominance Exam. Screens for mixed dominance or evidence that a person may have differences in hand, eye, and leg preferences that can signal neurological concerns

the neurological crossover that occurs in the body, problems with the functioning on the left side of the body would suggest right-hemisphere dysfunction.

Tests of Social/Behavioral Functioning

To assist in the process of diagnosing AS at least two measures have been developed. The Australian Scale for Asperger's Syndrome (ASAS), developed by M. S. Garnett and Tony Attwood, is a parent-completed rating-scale questionnaire covering commonly observed behaviors in children with AS. The Gilliam Asperger's Disorder Scale (GADS) is a parent-interview measure that asks about developmental and behavioral concerns consistent with AS.

The Child's Behavior Checklist (CBCL) and the Behavior Assessment System for Children (BASC) are two tests that use parent reports to look for clusters of concerns such as anxiety, depression, attention problems, aggressive behaviors, and social skill difficulties. For children with NLD and AS, we typically see elevations on the anxiety index, as well as on those that indicate attention problems, social skill weaknesses, and sometimes depression (especially in kids from ten to eighteen).

Although few social skills tests have been devised in general, the ASAS and the GADS tap into several of the areas in which children with AS or NLD struggle. We have also used apperception tests, such as the Roberts Apperception Test, informally as measures of social reasoning and the capacity to read social cues.

Preparing for an NLD or AS Evaluation

To prepare your child for this evaluation, it is usually helpful to talk about the testing as a way to understand how he learns best. Once we know that, we can help his teachers work with him in the ways that are most suitable for him, hopefully helping him learn more easily and making school more enjoyable. Usually, kids with suspected NLD or AS will be at least somewhat aware of their academic struggles in math, writing, organization, and understanding what they read. Depending on the child, he may or may not understand that he also has social skill weaknesses. You may want to say that the evaluation will also help us to understand why it is hard for him to make friends and to find ways to help him do so in the future. It is possible that your child will feel nervous about the evaluation, as it is new and unfamiliar to him. Telling him about the appointment ahead of time, but not too far in advance, may make him more comfortable, as will explaining how it will be "kind of fun" and really helpful to him.

Because the tasks that are usually rather fun for kids (puzzles, drawing, blocks) during a neuropsychological evaluation tend to be difficult for children with AS or NLD, a good evaluator will find other ways to make the session enjoyable and positive. Using praise and pointing out your child's strengths will be important during the evaluation; it is also useful to have a reward of some kind promised at the end of the session (e.g., a small toy/prize, going out for an ice cream cone, etc.).

The Testing's Completed: Now What Do I Do?

If your child is diagnosed with either NLD or AS after a thorough, comprehensive neuropsychological evaluation, there are a number of things that you can do as a parent to help him. First, read the sidebar "Things to Keep in Mind after You Receive the Report" in Chapter Six. Know that follow-up evaluations are often recommended, including a full speech and language evaluation and an occupational therapy and sensory integration evaluation. These should be available through your public school system, and you will be able to document the need for the tests with your special education department so that the department will provide these evaluations at no cost to you (see Chapter Two for the how-tos on this). Sometimes consultation with a neurologist, a medical doctor specializing in the brain and nervous system, is recommended. It is typically a good idea to follow through on these recommended evaluations, as they tend to provide additional information about your child that assists you and the school in designing an optimal education plan for him.

Treatment

Though we will not attempt to describe in detail the types of teaching and services recommended for children with NLD and AS—these are covered well by sources recommended at the end of this chapter and at the back of the book—the following interventions are typically considered to be necessary components of an IEP for this population:

What Should I Tell My Child about the Diagnosis?

Because most kids are relieved to find out that their problems actually have a name and that a lot of other kids have similar concerns, we generally recommend that you and/or the psychologist working with your child talk to him about the diagnosis. It's important to use age-appropriate explanations that will help him understand himself better rather than become more confused. Talk about his strengths first: "We learned that you are super great at reading words and spelling." "You know so many facts about space and dinosaurs—a lot more than kids your age usually know." Then follow with a brief explanation of the concerns: "You know how math has been getting harder for you? Well, all kids with a nonverbal learning disorder have trouble with math, too, but now we know how to help your teachers work with you better." "Kids with Asperger's usually have trouble figuring out what other people are thinking and feeling, so we're going to work on that with Ms. James at school." Be sure to convey the hopefulness that exists because we have many resources and interventions available now. You, too, should find information and support using the resources listed at the end of the chapter and by looking on-line for area groups.

- A low student–teacher ratio or an available aide
- Occupational therapy or sensory integration therapy
- Speech and language therapy, including pragmatics
- Physical therapy for gross-motor coordination and strength
- Keyboarding instruction
- Use of educational computer software to enhance skills where weaknesses exist
- Social skills training in a small group
- Social skills facilitation throughout the school day
- Class accommodations provided for children with ADHD (see Chapter Seven)
- Organization tutoring
- Special education services as needed in reading comprehension, math, and written expression
- Clear, concise information about assignments and tests
- A schedule or routine, with advance notice of any necessary changes

- Overt and clear bridges between new and old information and concepts, reinforced often
- Use of areas of interest as a means of fostering self-esteem, involvement in community activities, small interest groups, and so forth.
- Work with the school psychologist or outside mental health clinician on social reasoning, anxiety reduction and relaxation, understanding feelings
- Often (but not always) a medication consultation with a neurologist or child psychiatrist to address issues with attention, rigidity, mood, anxiety, and clarity of thinking (e.g., paranoid thinking)

One of the primary interventions that you can provide for your child is educating yourself about NLD or AS. You are then in a much better position to advocate for your child while having more patience for and understanding of his behavior. Sharing key articles or chapters on these concerns with your child's team at school is critical, especially if they are not particularly knowledgeable or familiar with NLD or AS. Then you will literally and figuratively be on the same page regarding your child and will be able to give him the educational support that he needs to be his best.

Resources

Books for Parents

Attwood, T. (1998). *Asperger's syndrome: A guide for parents and professionals.* London: Jessica Kingsley.

Ayres, J. (1979). *Sensory integration and the child.* Los Angeles, CA: Western Psychological Services.

Bashe, P., et al. (2001). *The OASIS guide to Asperger syndrome: Advice, support, insight, and inspiration.* New York: Crown.

Kranowitz, C. S. (1998). *The out of sync child: Recognizing and coping with sensory integration dysfunction.* New York: Perigree.

Nowicki, S., & Duke, M. P. (1992). *Helping the child who doesn't fit in.* Atlanta, GA: Peachtree.

Ozonoff, S., Dawson, G., & McPartland, J. (2002). *A parent's guide to Asperger Syndrome and high-functioning autism.* New York: Guilford Press.

Stewart, K. (2002). *Helping a child with nonverbal learning disorder or Asperger's Syndrome.* Oakland, CA: New Harbinger.

Whitney, R. (2002). *Bridging the gap: Raising a child with nonverbal learning disorder.* New York: Perigree.

Organizations/Web Sites

Asperger Syndrome Coalition of the United States (ASC-US)
P.O. Box 49267
Jacksonville Beach, FL 32240
www.asperger.org

Nonverbal Learning Disorders Association (NLDA)
999 Asylum Avenue
Hartford, CT 06105
www.nlda.org

Nonverbal Learning Disorder Online
www.nldline.com

Online Asperger's Syndrome Information and Support (OASIS)
www.aspergersyndrome.org

TAWK: Talking as a Way of Knowing (Nonverbal Learning Disorder)
www.nldsupport.org

Nine

Autism and Pervasive Developmental Disorder

Autism and its less-discussed cousin, pervasive developmental disorder (PDD), are *developmental disorders* that have essentially the same core features: delays in language and communication skills, impaired social skills, difficulty with symbolic play and imagination, and problems developing a *theory of mind*. The terms are sometimes used interchangeably, and we have seen kids with reports from physicians that say the diagnosis is "autism/PDD." This diagnosis is somewhat understandable, as the conditions lie along a continuum and the line between the two can sometimes seem rather arbitrary. Kids who are given the PDD label, however, tend either to be less impaired than fully autistic children or to have most but not all of the primary signs of autism.

We met Alexandria back in Chapter One, when her parents had begun to be concerned about her lack of interest in other kids. At first they thought the reason was that she was an only child, but soon it be-

---

Developmental disorders are understood as originating at birth or prenatally and typically affect the child across several domains, such as language, motor, and/or social skills. It is also generally understood that the disorder-associated problems will continue throughout the person's life, though treatment is often effective in reducing the severity of the delays.

Theory of mind is essentially the ability to recognize that others have thoughts and experiences that may be different from yours. It also involves being able to take another person's perspective, which is the basis for empathy, an important social skill.

came clear that she was quite different from other three-year-olds. Not only did she have trouble making eye contact and communicating well with words; she often did strange things like flapping her arms when she was stressed or excited. She played a lot on her own, usually reenacting scenes from her favorite video. After having Alexandria tested, her parents learned that she had something called *pervasive developmental disorder*, which was related to autism but generally not as severe. They also found out that, like other kids with PDD, Alexandria needed a lot of services immediately to address her delays in language, social skills, and motor skills.

The word *autistic* actually means "of the self," and this is perhaps the most striking feature of autistic children—they at least initially appear to be very much in their own world. Starting in infancy, autistic babies often fail to initiate social interaction via smiling or reaching their arms out to be held as other babies do. Some have a symptom called *tactile defensiveness*, a type of sensory processing disturbance that causes gentle caresses to be experienced as uncomfortable or even painful. Infants with autism therefore often arch their backs, stiffen, or cry when cuddled.

> **Tactile defensiveness** is an aspect of sensory integration dysfunction that involves a heightened sensitivity to touch, causing certain contact to be experienced as uncomfortable or even painful.

As they become toddlers and preschoolers, the deficits in language and communication, social interaction, and play skills become more obvious. It is usually between ages two and five that autism and PDD are first diagnosed. Some autistic children begin to use words and then experience a plateau or loss of language. This symptom is also seen in at least two other childhood disorders usually included in the category of developmental disorders, Rett syndrome and childhood disintegrative disorder. It is important to consider these as possible diagnoses if the child has lost language and other previously acquired skills, such as bowel/bladder training, motor skills such as picking up small objects or drawing, and social skills such as eye contact or interactive play.

What causes autism? We aren't yet sure, but we are certain that currently we are observing a surge in its occurrence. Research has indicated that multiple genes seem to be involved but do not seem to be the only factors causing the disorder to arise. If they were, then the identical twin of an autistic child would have a 100 percent chance of also having autism; as it stands, the research has found that chance to be only about 60 percent. There is certainly something going on genetically, though, because families with one autistic child are much more likely to have another autistic child or one with some autistic features.

Such things as environmental toxins, prenatal complications, and birth trauma have been suspected as causes of autism, as have allergies, immunological deficiencies, and metabolic problems in the child himself. Because a small number of children seemed to develop autism after they received the measles–mumps–rubella vaccine, a large-scale study looking into the possibility that this vaccine may cause or bring out autism has been initiated through the Centers for Disease Control and Prevention (CDC) and the National Institutes of Health (NIH). The smaller studies and reviews done so far, though, have *not* found any causal links between the vaccine and autism.

As we mentioned, the statistics for autism, PDD, and another developmental disorder, Asperger syndrome, have skyrocketed over the past few years. Currently, it is estimated that there are more than one million children and adults with autism in the United States, making these disorders five times more common than Down syndrome. As noted in recent popular media sources such as *Time* and *Wired* magazines, California alone has experienced an increase of over 200 percent in the rate of autistic children seeking services, from about four thousand in 1987 to now over 18,000. Though a rise in children diagnosed and seeking services for autism may be due in part to better detection, this disorder has not been thought to have been grossly overlooked in the past, as the symptoms are fairly obvious. So it looks as if there has been a real increase in the number of children with autism over the past several years. If your child has a developmental disorder, the good news for you is that the growing demand for services is bound to make them more readily available and higher in quality.

Diagnosing Autism and Pervasive Developmental Disorder

Although the diagnosis of autism or PDD is typically given between ages two and five, there are some earlier red flags, including the lack of social interaction or interest in others—such as not smiling or holding arms out—discussed previously. Though it is typical for children to begin babbling and pointing to things by age one, an autistic child often fails to do so. By age two, he may not be using any words, although at least two-word phrases should be emerging. We also expect two-year-olds to be imitating others as a form of learning and interacting, but the autistic child usually does not do so. Early on, the child shows a lack of responsiveness when the child's name is called and an absence of pretend, or symbolic, play. Three-year-old Christopher reportedly "played" with his dinosaur figures, but upon closer observation it became clear that he was simply lining them up or watching them fall from the table to the floor over and over. In this section we look at each of the core features of autism and PDD, which include significant delays in social skills, communication, play skills, and certain cognitive skills such as theory of mind and executive functions, giving you more specifics to go by. If you should notice more than two of the behaviors in each category, we strongly recommend you talk with your pediatrician.

Social Interaction

Often from infancy but almost always by age three, parents of autistic children report that they simply seemed "in their own world" or at least not very interested in or attuned to things going on around them. They often show a preference for being alone and a tendency to become stressed or anxious when people try to engage them. Little to no effort to greet others is made, and if it is, it's usually through awkward or inappropriate means. Affected kids do not always seek comfort and may have trouble knowing when or how to provide it to others. Many researchers believe this behavior is linked to the autistic child's lack of theory of mind, or difficulty in understanding another's perspective. This is the root of empathy, as well as social reasoning skills; children with autism and PDD are therefore at a great disadvantage without this essential ability.

That said, we have known many autistic children who are quite affectionate and quick to comfort others in their own unique way. Ten-year-old Charlotte loved to be cuddled by her mom, especially when she felt anxious or tired. Seven-year-old Terry knew that his younger brother's tears meant he needed attention, and he would go over and pat his back (sometimes a little too hard, but that's okay). In light of our experience and that of other professionals we know, we caution readers in assuming that autistic children aren't capable of connecting or even loving others; in fact, they can and do routinely.

Language/Communication Skills

Although most autistic children will eventually acquire at least some language skills, these skills are commonly delayed and impaired. They usually have difficulty both understanding what is said (receptive language skills) and verbalizing their ideas and needs (expressive language skills). Autistic children often sound odd when they speak; their manner of speaking can sound mechanical, repetitive, too loud, or monotone. They also tend to place the emphasis on the wrong words, giving their speech a noticeably unusual quality.

Echolalia is another common feature of autistic children's speech. Literally, they echo what others say. During an evaluation of six-year-old Stan, who hadn't said a word in more than half an hour, he must have somehow been intrigued by the comment "That was awesome, Stan!" And so, for the next hour or more, he uttered this four-word sentence at least twenty times. Amanda, a four-year-old with autism, frequently quoted from her favorite children's video, sometimes several lines at a time. It's important to realize that the meaning and use of the verbal information is often lost on the child, so echolalia can give the false impression that the child has more language capacity than he actually has. Likewise, many autistic children learn to decode words when they read but struggle significantly with understanding what the words mean (reading comprehension).

Problems with social communication, sometimes called *pragmatics,* are common for children with autism and PDD, too. Eye contact is a very common problem area. When they want to initiate interaction with someone, autistic children either avoid eye contact altogether or use it fleetingly or too intensely. Whereas typical children learn to read and understand social cues such as facial expressions or gestures gradually as they mature, those with autism and PDD often find these abilities elusive even when grown up.

Play Skills

By about age two and a half, the autism-associated deficits in play skills really begin to stand out. Specifically, the play of children with autism and PDD tends to be qualitatively different, failing to reflect an ability to use toys in a symbolic way. To the autistic child, a block is just a block rather than having the potential to be a boat, a building, or a car. Rather than using figures to play out an imagined scenario, the autistic child's version of this type of play may be to use figures to exactly replicate a scene observed on television. One little boy seen in our office could enact an entire thirty-minute dinosaur video but never strayed from the script and could not allow others to join in the activity. Autistic kids often spend hours lining up toys, flipping one piece of a toy over and over, or engaging in some other similar repetitive activity.

Other Common Features

The majority of children diagnosed with autism or PDD will demonstrate impaired executive functions, including difficulty "shifting gears," organization problems, impulsivity, and very short attention spans. (More detailed information on executive functions can be found in Chapter Seven.) Sometimes affected kids will tune out for a few seconds or more routinely and will seem to go somewhere else in their minds. For some autistic children, this behavior signals absence seizures, or irregular brain activity that causes a disturbance in the child's capacity to function for a brief period of time. Children with autism are at a higher risk for seizure disorders, and electroencephalograms (EEGs) or other tests are often performed to determine whether or not seizures are occurring. If they are, the seizures are usually well controlled with medication.

Autistic children also tend to have sensory processing and integration problems, which were discussed in the previous chapter. Tactile hypersensitivity, or a strong reaction to touch and textures in clothes and food, is common, as is auditory hypersensitivity (oversensitivity to sound). Sensory integration dysfunction, the diagnosis given when many sensory systems are affected, is frequently diagnosed in children with autism and PDD.

Repetitive movements such as rocking or flapping are also common in children with these developmental disorders. These behaviors are considered to be a source of self-stimulation, or a means of creating a certain level of arousal that is otherwise too low or too high. Autistic children seem to use these actions to soothe or calm themselves as well, because there tends to be an increase in self-stimulatory behaviors (called *stimming*) when affected kids are stressed or anxious.

Though children with autism and PDD tend to have adequate or even advanced gross-motor coordination, we often see problems with fine-motor skills. Writing, using scissors, and tying shoelaces, for example, may be extra challenging for this population.

What the Testing Evaluation Should Include

Although pediatricians, neurologists, and other professionals may be able to accurately diagnose a child with autism or PDD without the assistance of testing, it is generally routine to refer these patients for a developmental, educational, or neuropsychological evaluation, as well as speech and language assessments and occupational therapy and sensory integration evaluations. The results provide a general guide for parents, teachers, and therapists with respect to the child's level of need, optimal learning style, and potential to reach a certain level of skill.

Q: *In the parents' group that I'm in, several mothers talk about the behavior problems of their autistic children. One child has severe tantrums in which he will even bite and punch his family members. So far, my son doesn't seem to have this type of problem. How common is it, and what can I do about it if my son starts doing this kind of thing?*

A: Although on the whole children with autism or PDD are not violent, behavior problems that include frequent tantrums, problems with emotional lability, and aggression directed at others and themselves (e.g., head banging) are fairly common. Fortunately, many behavior programs have been developed for kids with autism, but depending on where you live, the availability varies greatly. Applied behavioral analysis (ABA) and the Lovaas Method place a strong emphasis on behavior modification, but these are actually comprehensive programs designed to address most of the concerns related to autism, not just the behavioral issues. Because of this, these programs can be expensive and are usually quite time-consuming, too. Getting involved through parent groups, autism advocacy groups, research on-line, and involvement in the school system may help you locate the appropriate program for your child should he develop any behavior problems. You should also talk with the clinicians involved with your child, such as his speech and language therapist or occupational therapist, for strategies and resources for behavior management, as well as social skills training.

Emotional lability refers to highly variable emotional states—one minute the child may be content, and the next he is yelling in frustration.

As part of your child's evaluation, you will need to provide a full history and will likely here to complete some behavioral assessment forms such as the ABC (Autism Behavior Checklist), the WADIC (Wing Autistic Disorder Interview Checklist), or the CHAT (Checklist for Autism in Toddlers). We recommend that your child at least attempt to complete the following tests as part of a thorough educational and neuropsychological evaluation.

Developmental Measures

For children four and under, it is often helpful to receive a developmental assessment using interview, observation, and a measure such as the Bayley Scales of Infant Development, the Denver Developmental Screening Test, the BRIGANCE screens, or the Child Development Inventories. These tests give you a sense of how far outside the range of "normal" your child may fall with respect to skills in language, motor ability, social ability, and cognition.

Intelligence Testing

Although intelligence test results can be quite variable among these kids, it is fairly common to find that autistic children have lower verbal IQ scores than Performance or nonverbal IQ scores, given the extent of the language impairment they tend to experience. On the WISC-IV, many children with autism or PDD will demonstrate a "splinter skill," an area of marked strength, on the Block Design subtest. This test involves copying designs with red and white blocks, tapping a child's abstract visual–spatial skills and constructional abilities.

We caution parents and clinicians alike, though, when reading the results of intelligence testing in particular, because generally the most commonly used IQ measures, such as the WISC-IV and the DAS, end up underestimating the autistic child's true potential. These tests rely heavily on language skills, fine-motor skills, and attention skills—three typical areas of weakness for children with autism and PDD. Seven-year-old Steven, for example, was asked to tell what the word *watch* meant on an intelligence test. Because of his language impairment, the best he could do was to say "clock"; although his answer suggested that he had the concept of what a watch was and could do, he could not get credit for his response. This is the type of concern we are speaking about when we ask readers to interpret intelligence test results of autistic children with care, particularly because the results may lead you to significantly underestimate your child's potential to do all sorts of things.

Tests such as the TONI-3, a test of nonverbal intelligence that does not require language skills, are suggested given that they may provide a more accurate measure of an autistic child's potential. Still, the novelty of the testing situation, which can be stressful to these kids, and variable attention often interfere with optimal performance.

Achievement/Educational Testing

This type of testing also should be given if your child is of school age. Many children with autism and PDD learn to read well but have trouble understanding the meaning of the information they read (reading comprehension). Sometimes math is an area of strength, but problems arise when the concepts become more abstract. Writing skills are typically weak, but using the computer to facilitate written work and communication in general has been quite successful.

Language Tests

It is routine for a child with autism or PDD to see a speech and language therapist for a full evaluation. During a neuropsychological evaluation, psychologists may use tests such as the Boston Naming Test, the Expressive One-Word Vocabulary Test, and the Peabody Picture Vocabulary Test to assess the child's basic expressive and receptive language skills.

Visual–Spatial/Visual–Motor Skills

Although we generally recommend a full occupational therapy evaluation, which examines these types of skills, as well as others, it is common for a neuropsychological evaluation to include several measures related to these skills. The nonverbal subtests of intelligence tests, such as the WISC-IV Block Design and Matrix Reasoning, are commonly given, as are measures such as the Developmental Test of Visual–Motor Integration.

Executive-Function-Based Tests

We recommend that the evaluator you are working with administer tests such as the Wide Range Assessment of Memory and Learning (WRAML), Trails A and B, the Children's Category Test, and the California Verbal Learning Test for Children. On the measures of sustained auditory attention, shifting set ("shifting gears"), and complex problem solving, we would expect the majority of children with autism and PDD to perform relatively poorly. Scores on tasks that assess visual attention and rote memory skills (visual and verbal) are often better.

Sensorimotor and Neuromotor Tests

Again, a thorough occupational therapy evaluation will examine these functions, but often a full neuropsychological assessment will include tests such as Finger Tapping, Grooved Pegboard, and Lateral Dominance Exam to examine the child's motor output, strength, and any right–left differences that may exist.

Tests of Social and Behavioral Functioning

In addition to a specific autism-related measure such as the ones mentioned earlier, the ABC or the CHAT, you may be asked to complete general behavior scales such as the Child Behavior Checklist (CBCL) or the Behavior Assessment System for Children (BASC). The evaluation should also include clinical observations of your child's behavior and social functioning, which should be written up in the report under a heading such as "Behavioral Observations" or "Behavioral/Social Functioning."

Preparing for an Autism Evaluation

Children who are suspected of having autism or PDD are typically referred for a developmental or neuropsychological evaluation, a speech and language evaluation, and an occupational therapy evaluation. Although the public school can provide aspects of the evaluations described previously, you should know that you can obtain private evaluations with clinicians who specialize in developmental disorders. On the whole, affected kids are difficult to test using regular methods, and often the parents are asked to help out during the testing process.

Q: *My pediatrician says you can't diagnose autism in a child younger than two years of age. Is that true? If not, how can testing help?*

A: Some people believe that because there is such variability in normal development it is difficult or poor practice to diagnose developmental disorders such as autism in very young children. However, more recent research and new measures such as the CHAT (Checklist for Autism in Toddlers) and the CHAT-M (a modified version) have helped make the distinction between slightly lagging skills and true delays that are characteristic of autism or PDD. This measure, coupled with a good history, play observation, and a developmental test such as the Bayley or the BRIGANCE, should allow accurate detection and diagnosis in children as young as eighteen months. This is very important, as we have found that the earlier you intervene, the better the child typically does.

Q: *Our daughter was diagnosed with high-functioning autism (HFA) by a pediatric neurologist. When we looked on-line, we found that a lot of sources say that HFA and Asperger syndrome (AS) are the same thing. The psychologist who did the testing evaluation with our daughter, though, said that these are really two different but related disorders. Who is right?*

A: We can't claim to know the answer to this one, especially as the field is in great debate about this issue. What we *can* tell you from experience, as well as information from the Yale Child Study Center, is that there does seem to be a true distinction between HFA and AS, primarily in the extent of the language skill impairment. People with HFA tend to have weaker receptive (ability to understand) and expressive (ability to verbalize thoughts, needs, etc.) language skills than people with AS. Often on intelligence testing, then, children with HFA will have lower verbal IQ scores than Performance/nonverbal IQ scores. This is the exact reverse of what we tend to see in kids with AS, as they typically have lower Performance IQ scores.

To prepare your child for the evaluation, tell him that he will be going to a new place to do some fun things with Ms. or Mr. So-and-So; using the term "doctor" may cause unnecessary distress, and affected kids may be able to associate this term only with shots and other discomforts. It will be important for you to take along favorite toys, foods and snacks, and books to use during breaks and for calming. If your child has a tough time separating from you or performs poorly in new situations, you should talk with the evaluator about sitting in on the session. Often, parents are a great help in assisting the evaluator and informing her about skills or weaknesses that were not evident during the testing. You may be asked to interpret questions for your child using language he is familiar with to get the most accurate read on his skills. Likewise, you may need to help the evaluator understand what your child is trying to communicate verbally or nonverbally. You can anticipate several brief testing periods with many breaks, though the whole evaluation may occur in one day. We strongly suggest having some sort of treat or reward ready that can be used to motivate your child during the evaluation. Try not to feel too discouraged if your child seems to be having a lot of trouble performing on the tests; a psychologist specializing in developmental disorders will know how to glean useful information about your child's abilities regardless of how many answers he gets right.

The Testing's Completed: Now What Do I Do?

Our guess is that once you receive the diagnosis of autism or PDD for your child, you will feel a mixture of relief and despair. The relief may come from finally having a way to understand the concerns you've had about your child, as well as from knowing that a lot can be done to help. (These interventions should be discussed in the Recommendations section of the evaluation report; see the sidebar "Things to Keep in Mind after You Receive the Report" in Chapter Six.) You may feel despair, though, as you find that your dreams of a "normal" life for you and your child seem impossible. Because of these feelings, we can't stress enough the importance of connecting with other families who have children with developmental disorders. You will likely find your hope restored as you hear success stories and learn about additional therapies and resources now available to help your child.

Treatment

Fortunately, a wealth of research on autism and PDD has helped us treat these disorders more effectively. The best approach is a multifac-

What Should I Tell My Child about the Diagnosis?

For the most part, children diagnosed with autism will have trouble understanding even brief, simple explanations of the disorder. Kids with less severe forms of PDD should be informed about their diagnosis to the extent that it helps them understand why they need to go see so many teachers or helpers at school and how they will get better at things such as talking, jumping, and making friends if they keep going and trying. Involvement in social skills groups with other children who have PDD or autism will likely be helpful in showing them that they're not alone. You, too, will benefit from a parents' group in your area, as this is often the best place to get information about resources, programs, and behavior management, as well as support and encouragement.

eted one, with many different care providers and services working toward the common goal of helping your child interact with the world more successfully.

Your public school system can be your main ally in that all services may be coordinated through your child's team and/or by contracting out to area specialists for the services the school system should provide but cannot. The diagnoses of autism and PDD tend to convey to school systems a significant level of care and need. However, we've seen incredible variability with respect to the services and programs offered to children with these diagnoses. Of course, the kids themselves vary widely in severity of impairments and behavioral issues, but generally children with autism and PDD should get the following services at school and home:

- If younger than age three, Early Intervention (EI) services for speech and language
- Occupational therapy, behavior therapy, and social skill development several times per week
- A structured language-based program that relies heavily on multisensory instruction for school-age children
- A specialized placement in a program specifically for students with autism or developmental disorders (for children with se-

vere autism or those living in a school system with few resources)

- Intensive speech and language therapy (usually at least three to five times a week)
- Intensive occupational therapy for fine-motor skills and sensory integration
- Behavioral therapy or a program to address concerns such as self-stimulation, inattention, tantrums, aggression, socialization, and so forth
- Social skill facilitation in small structured groups, as well as throughout the day
- A one-to-one trained aide (if in a mainstream setting) for activities or classes
- After-school and/or home-based services for behavior and social skills
- Summer services provided by the school system for speech and language therapy
- Occupational therapy, social skills facilitation, and educational support to prevent skill regression over the summer vacation
- Consultation with an allergist or dietician to determine whether food allergies (e.g., to dairy or wheat) may be contributing to your child's symptoms
- Consultation with a pediatric neurologist who may recommend follow-up tests such as EEGs and genetic testing
- Medication evaluation with a specializing child psychiatrist or neurologist (selective serotonin reuptake inhibitors [SSRIs] and at times stimulants have proven very helpful to kids with PDD)
- Parent support groups, sibling support groups, and other resources for the family, such as books, Web sites, and conferences

As with many things, the earlier and more intensive the interventions for children with these developmental disorders, the better. It may be tempting to eliminate services for kids as they show progress, but doing so typically leads to a loss of or plateau in skill development. Updating your child's evaluation in all areas (speech and language, occupational therapy and sensory integration, education evaluation, neuropsychological evaluation) about every two years is strongly recommended for monitoring purposes, as well as to support the need for continued services.

Resources

Books for Parents

Cohen, D. J., & Volkmar, F. R. (Eds.). (1997). *Handbook of autism and pervasive developmental disorders* (2nd ed.). New York: Wiley.

Hamilton, L., & Rimland, B. (1999). *Facing autism: Giving parents reasons for hope and guidance for help.* New York: Waterbrook Press.

Hart, C. (1993). *Parent's guide to autism.* New York: Pocket Books.

Kranowitz, C. S. (1998). *The out of sync child: Recognizing and coping with sensory integration dysfunction.* New York: Perigree.

Seroussi, K. (2002). *Unraveling the mystery of autism and pervasive developmental disorder.* New York: Broadway Books.

Organizations/Web Sites

Autism Resources
www.autism-info.com

Autism Society of America
7910 Woodmont Avenue, Suite 650
Bethesda, MD 20814
www.autism-society.org

Families for Early Autism Treatment
www.feat.org

Yale Child Study Center
info.med.yale.edu/chldstdy/autism

Ten

Mathematics Disorder and Disorder of Written Expression

Children who have specific learning disabilities in math and/or writing obviously can have great difficulty succeeding in school. Unfortunately, much less is known about these two disorders than about other disorders we've reviewed in this book, in part because they seem to affect a comparatively small number of children. Mathematics disorder without co-occurring dyslexia, nonverbal learning disability, or another related problem has been estimated to affect only about 1 percent of school-age children. We think that disorder of written expression, particularly when it occurs alone, is even rarer, though we don't know if that's the case because we lack good estimates of prevalence.

What we do know is that these disorders have several features in common. First, a person's ability in either of these areas, as measured on standardized tests, is substantially lower than we'd expect based on age, education, and intelligence. Second, these difficulties impede the child's ability in academic achievement or activities of daily living. Third, if the child also has a sensory deficit, such as in visual perception, memory, or attention, the difficulties in math or writing are worse than what would be expected with the sensory deficit alone. If a child with a math disorder has attentional difficulties, for example, his difficulties in math will be worse than what we'd expect from a child with attentional difficulties. Fourth, individualized testing is always necessary to make either diagnosis.

Children with math and writing problems tend to be diagnosed later than children with dyslexia, ADHD, Asperger syndrome, or nonverbal learning disorder, probably because their difficulties don't affect their classroom performance in the early school years. Math and written expression are not as large a part of the school curriculum as reading is during early elementary school. Problems in math or writing do not have pervasive effects on functioning, as problems with inattention or hyperactivity do. However, the school environment has changed much over the past decade, and the amount of written output a child is asked to produce has increased. As a result, writing problems (including both the physical act of writing and problems with other aspects of writing, such as organizing thoughts, generating ideas, and translating ideas to a written form) are having an impact earlier in a child's educational history than we saw in the past.

Mathematics Disorder

Sharon was a typical fourth grader in every way but one—she had incredible difficulty with math. Although she was a good reader and speller, she became very frustrated during math class. Word problems were the worst. Her teacher and parents were at a loss as to what to do. Sharon appeared to understand the lessons in school but couldn't remember how to use what she'd learned by the time she sat down to do her homework. At other times she seemed prepared for a math test (as when she studied with her dad the night before) but then failed the test. When her dad tried to help her with her homework by having her draw a picture of the concepts, Sharon had no idea how to do it. Her parents brought her into our clinic because she began saying things like "I'm dumb. I can't learn anything." Sharon had many other positive attributes—she was a good athlete who had many friends, for example—but her problems with math seemed to be damaging her self-esteem. Her parents also wondered if Sharon might not be trying hard enough, so they sought an evaluation to clarify the nature of her difficulties.

Sharon's presentation is a typical one for a child with a math disorder. She showed a fairly normal development until second or third grade, when math concepts became hard for her to learn. Sharon also demonstrated difficulty learning to tell time and learning about money. What confused her parents and teacher most of all was that Sharon had no idea when her answers to math problems were right or wrong. Her answers to problems were sometimes wildly incorrect. For example, when asked to solve the problem "50 x 100," she wrote *105*. When asked what a reasonable answer to this question might be, she was unable to say.

Sharon's test results indicated that she had higher verbal than nonverbal IQ scores, with a Full Scale IQ in the average range. Tests of oral reading, spelling, and reading comprehension were slightly above grade level. Tests of visual–spatial ability were in the low-average range. Tests of math ability were at the 1.8 grade level. Neuropsychological tests indicated that Sharon had weaknesses in executive functions, particularly on tests that required flexibility in thinking and higher level abstract thinking.

In terms of her performance on the math achievement tests, Sharon often misunderstood the mathematical operation she was asked to perform. For example, she initially responded to the problem "4 – 3 =" with the answer "7" and to the problem "10 + 3 =" with the answer "7." It wasn't just a question of her misreading the signs, because when her incorrect answers were pointed out to her, it often took her more than one try to answer the question correctly. For example, when she was told her answer to "4 – 3 = 7" was incorrect, she changed her answer to "12," stating that she multiplied 4 and 3. Although she had the basic math facts memorized, she wasn't able to apply them because she didn't have a good mastery of the concepts.

Once the testing was completed, a number of recommendations were suggested for Sharon. First, tutoring in math was recommended. Sharon needed help in figuring out how to "attack" a math problem, as well as help in learning the conceptual aspects of math. The evaluator suggested that the tutor and classroom teacher make use of concrete "manipulatives," such as Cuisenaire rods and

> **Dyscalculia** means an inability to calculate and is often used interchangeably with *mathematics disorder.*

that Sharon be provided with "recipes" for solving multistep problems such as long division. She also needed to be taught such strategies as estimating her answers in advance. These suggestions were effective in helping Sharon achieve more success in math.

Diagnosing Mathematics Disorder

As mentioned previously, formal, individualized testing is necessary to make a diagnosis of mathematics disorder. It is difficult to make this diagnosis until a child reaches school age, however, because the child's progress in math must be below age, grade, and intellectual expectations. Sometimes warning signs can be found in a child's history, such as poor sense of direction, poor athletic coordination, difficulty keeping score in board games, problems learning strategic games such as chess, and difficulty learning abstract concepts such as time or money.

Unfortunately, these types of evaluations are not usually covered by most insurance companies. A typical comprehensive evaluation will cost $1,200 to $2,500 or more. Your child can be tested through the school district at no cost to you. The school won't typically diagnose your child with a learning disability but will determine whether her achievement is significantly discrepant from her intellectual abilities. If so, the school will provide whatever services it deems appropriate. (See Chapter Two for more information on how to obtain an evaluation through your local school district.) If an actual diagnosis is important to you, you'll probably need to have your child evaluated by an independent psychologist.

What the Testing Evaluation Should Include

A developmental history is important, but it does not provide enough information to make a diagnosis. A comprehensive evaluation would include:

- An interview with the parent and child that includes information about developmental and educational history.
- A test of intelligence, such as the Wechsler Intelligence Scale for Children (WISC-IV), Stanford–Binet, or Differential Ability Scales (DAS)
- Tests of academic achievement, such as the Woodcock–Johnson, Wide Range Achievement Test (WRAT), or Wechsler Individual Achievement Test (WIAT-II)
- Neuropsychological tests are also often given, par-

IQ-achievement discrepancy refers to academic performance that is markedly lower than would be expected based on a child's intellectual ability.

ticularly tests of executive functions and visual–motor and spatial abilities.

We would expect children with a math disability to have scores that were selectively low in math, most often by demonstrating an IQ-achievement and/or grade–achievement discrepancy on standardized tests. Some of the more commonly used tests of math achievement include:

WIAT-II Subtests

- *Numerical Operations.* On this subtest, the child is presented with a math work sheet and asked to solve problems. Younger children are asked to do things such as write dictated numbers or add and subtract one-digit numbers, and older students are asked to solve problems such as long division and algebra.
- *Math Reasoning.* This is a test of a child's ability to understand math concepts, such as geometric measurement, money, time, reading and interpreting graphs, and probability. Students are also asked to solve word problems that are read to them.

Woodcock–Johnson Tests of Achievement

- *Calculations.* On this subtest, children are presented with written math problems in a work sheet format that they are asked to solve.
- *Applied Problems.* This is a test of mathematical problem-solving ability, in which the child is read a story problem to solve or shown a graph to interpret.

Q: My five-year-old is in kindergarten. Are there any math tests that can be used to test a child this young?

A: The WIAT-II and Woodcock–Johnson tests mentioned previously can be used with children this young. Another is the Test of Early Mathematics Ability (TEMA-2). This test can be used with children ages three to eight and assesses concepts such as counting, the ability to match one item with another, and the ability to do simple arithmetic problems.

Differential Ability Scales

- *Basic Number Skills.* A written test of math problems

Wide Range Achievement Test

- *Math Subtest.* A written test of math problem-solving ability

In addition to tests of mathematical ability, tests of executive functions and spatial ability are often administered to help determine whether either of these areas underlie some of the difficulties a child might be experiencing. Some of the tests of executive functions that might be administered include those mentioned in Chapters 4 and 7:

> **Executive functions** are those abilities that allow an individual to plan, set goals, carry out goal-directed plans, and self-monitor behavior. (See Chapter Seven for more information.)

- *Wisconsin Card Sorting Test*
- *Trails A and B*

Other tests of executive functions could also include the:

- *Category Test.* A test requiring abstract concept formation and use of feedback information to form and test hypotheses.

Tests of spatial reasoning include the:

- Developmental Test of Visual–Motor Integration
- Rey–Osterrieth Complex Figure Test
- Bender Visual Motor Gestalt Test
- DAS Pattern Construction and Recall of Designs subtests
- WISC-IV Block Design or Matrix Reasoning subtests

Preparing for an Evaluation for Math Disorder

If you suspect your child has a learning disability in one of these areas, you'll want him to be evaluated by a licensed psychologist, such as a clinical psychologist, neuropsychologist, or school psychologist. A typical evaluation will take four to six hours. If your child is being evaluated

Q: My child's teacher said children with dyslexia often have trouble learning math facts, too. How do we know whether my son has dyslexia or a math disorder–or both?

A: The math problems that we see in children with dyslexia are different from those seen in children with a mathematics disorder. Children with dyslexia often have trouble memorizing math facts, such as multiplication tables. They also demonstrate difficulty in math when they are asked to solve story problems (because of their difficulty in reading the problems). Sometimes they have trouble writing numbers or reversing numbers. However, they do not typically have problems understanding math concepts. Children with a mathematics disorder can often memorize multiplication tables quite easily but have problems understanding the concepts that underlie mathematics or getting the "big picture."

It is possible, however, to have both disorders. It takes a trained clinician to determine whether a child with dyslexia who is having trouble in math meets criteria for a math disability or whether the difficulties in math can be attributed to the child's dyslexia.

Q: If the math problems can be attributed to dyslexia, does this mean the child doesn't need to receive special education services in math?

A: No, but the services the child receives might be quite different. For example, if a child with dyslexia is doing poorly in math because he can't read story problems, the treatment for that difficulty (help with reading the problems) is different from the treatment for a child with a math disorder (providing tutoring so that she understands how to solve the problem).

----

through his school, the evaluation will likely be scheduled over a number of test dates. If your child is being evaluated through a private clinic, he will likely be asked to come in for one or two test sessions.

To help your child understand what to expect, first let her know that you are having her tested so that you can find out how she learns best. Your child likely has an idea that certain aspects of school are not going well for her; therefore, let her know that you're concerned about her progress in math and that you want to know how to make things better for her. Second, let her know that she'll be spending a few hours with a doctor who will asking her to solve puzzles, do math problems, read, and draw, among other things. As we've stated before, most kids find the process quite fun, although tiring. Promise your child that you'll do something fun with her after she's done taking the tests.

You may be worried that your child may become uncooperative or distressed during this evaluation because the examiner will be evaluating her areas of weakness. However, the tests are not designed so that the child is continually confronted with problems she is unable to do. Instead, the child is generally first presented with problems that are easy for her. These problems get progressively more difficult. Once the child is unable to answer a certain number of problems, the examiner moves on to a different test. The math subtests are interspersed with others that measure different skills. In this way, the child isn't required to spend large periods of time being tested in her area of weakness. Thus problems with cooperation are rarely an issue if your child is seeing an experienced examiner.

The Testing's Completed: Now What Do I Do?

There is no single treatment program for all math disabilities, because the treatment depends on what the child's main deficits are. For example, one child's problems in math may be related to visual–spatial confusion, whereas another child's problems may be related to problems with getting the "big picture" or understanding the underlying concepts of mathematical problem solving. These children may have difficulties with executive functions and may see math as a collection of facts that need to be memorized. However, they have difficulty finding patterns and meaning in math. Other children have problems with all of these things. Determining which of these difficulties underlies a child's problem is extremely important—and the reason a battery of tests is necessary. The evaluation can define the areas of specific weakness so that individual tutoring (which is almost always recommended) can be custom designed. See the sidebar "Things to Keep in Mind after You Receive the Report" in Chapter Six for advice on taking the next step.

Treatment

Some approaches that are helpful for children include:

- Providing written "recipes" for complex math problems, such as long division
- Allowing the use of graph paper to help with aligning columns in written math problems

- Providing students with a more hands-on, concrete approach to learning math concepts, especially those that are spatial in nature
- Teaching children how to approach a problem or task, such as evaluating what operation is needed, learning to make a careful evaluation of whether the information in the problem is pertinent or nonessential, and estimating and checking answers against the estimate to evaluate their reasonableness
- Making math practically oriented, emphasizing things such as cooking and shopping so that children can see concretely the relevance of concepts such as decimals, fractions, and so forth

---

Q: Are there any strategies that are useful for high school and college students?

A: Many of the strategies for students at this age include providing tutoring as needed in particular subject areas (geometry, algebra, chemistry), as well as tailoring their course load to avoid their weaknesses and capitalize on their strengths. For example, if a child has difficulty with spatial abilities, geometry will be particularly difficult. In that case, if the child has a choice between geometry and algebra, it might be advisable to take algebra. Higher level math courses such as trigonometry and calculus will, in general, be quite difficult for a child with a math disability. Some of the science classes, particularly those that rely heavily on math ability, such as physics and chemistry, will also present challenges. In this case, students who have a choice regarding science credits might be better off taking science courses, such as biology or life science, that do not require mathematical skills.

Disorder of Written Expression

David was a good-natured sixth grader brought in for testing because he was having extreme difficulty completing homework and taking notes in school. His mother, Leslie, described David as a classic underachiever. She thought he was quite bright, but his schoolwork never reflected it. It was at Parents' Night in David's kindergarten class that she first wondered if David had a problem. On the bulletin board were self-portraits drawn by each of the students. As Leslie looked at the drawings, it was clear that David's were much poorer than the others. Whereas other children had decorated their self-portraits with flowers, trees, and detailed clothing, David's drawing consisted of a crudely drawn stick figure with a big smile on his face. Leslie and her husband, Bruce, laughingly noted that David would never be Picasso, but underneath her laughter Leslie wondered if something was wrong.

As David progressed through elementary school, his teachers constantly said that David just couldn't get through the work quickly enough. When presented with a work sheet, he often had trouble getting started, and he was almost always the last child in the classroom to complete his written work. It took him four times as long to complete his homework than it should have. Most notably, his work was always messy. Although David's teachers voiced their concerns, they ultimately told his parents not to worry, as David was one of the most well-liked children in class and one who actively participated in group discussions and class activities. However, David seemed to "hit a wall" when he started middle school in sixth grade, in which he was expected to take notes in every class, complete dozens of work sheets and study guides, and take timed essay tests. As a result, David's naturally happy disposition started to become one of frustration and sadness.

David's complaints and history were striking for his problems with written expression. In some ways he was lucky, because his strong social skills helped him compensate for his weaknesses in written expression. In other ways, he was at a disadvantage, because he was never given assistance to help remediate his problems.

David's test results indicated that his intelligence was in the above-average range, but his academic achievement ranged from low average on tasks of spelling and written expression to superior on tests of reading comprehension. Although his math achievement was near grade level, his performance was compromised by his poor written organizational skills (such as not lining up the columns correctly on multiplication and division problems). His spelling abilities were affected by the fact that he wrote words quickly and sloppily. It was very difficult to read what he had written. When the examiner asked him at one point, "What are these letters?" he couldn't tell her. On tests of visual–motor abilities, David did quite poorly, far below expectations for his grade and intellectual capabilities.

Once the testing was completed, we made a number of recommendations for David, such as that he be encouraged to type and provided with additional time to complete written work. We also recommended a reduction in written work when appropriate and assistance with note taking in class. We suggested that he receive an occupational therapy evaluation to determine whether additional treatment might be effective. Finally, we discussed the test results with David, who was quite amazed to know that he was as smart as, if not smarter than, many children in his class. We were able to talk to David about his disability and how that affected his ability to do his best. The evaluation enabled David and his family to reframe their image of him from one of a classic underachiever to one in which David was viewed as a bright child with severe difficulties with written expression.

Dysgraphia is a term that is often used interchangeably with disorder of written expression. The term means "an inability to write."

Diagnosing Disorder of Written Expression

An individualized assessment is necessary to make a diagnosis of disorder of written expression. It is rarely diagnosed before first or second grade because most children have not had sufficient formal writing instruction before that time. Sometimes, as in David's case, warning signs can be found in a child's history, such as poor drawing ability, a reluctance to do arts and crafts activities in preschool, difficulties with fine-motor skills, poor pencil grasp, and trouble learning to write letters. Sometimes the child's problem lies in an inability to come up with ideas or to get his ideas down on paper in an organized fashion. Many times we find that parents (especially parents of middle-school children) don't see their child as having problems with written output, but they see their child instead as being depressed, having low self-esteem, or being oppositional because he or she isn't completing schoolwork.

What the Testing Evaluation Should Include

Although a developmental history is important, more formal testing is necessary to make a diagnosis of disorder of written expression. A comprehensive evaluation would include:

- An interview with the parent and child that includes information about development and educational history
- A test of intelligence such as the Wechsler Intelligence Scale for Children (WISC-IV), Stanford–Binet, or Differential Ability Scales (DAS)

- Tests of academic achievement such as the Woodcock–Johnson, Wide Range Achievement Test (WRAT), or Wechsler Individual Achievement Test (WIAT-II)
- Tests of writing and visual motor abilities such as the Developmental Test of Visual–Motor Integration (VMI) and the Rey–Osterrieth (see Chapter Four)
- A writing sample, such as the Test of Written Language (TOWL)
- Sometimes tests of executive functions are given to rule out the possibility that attentional or organizational issues may be affecting a child's ability in written expression.

We would expect a child with a disorder of written expression to have scores that were selectively low on tests of written work and demonstrated an IQ–achievement and/or grade–achievement discrepancy on standardized tests. However, there are few standardized measures in this area, and as a result, qualitative observations, such as the neatness of the child's work, how the child holds a pencil, how automatic the child's writing is, and the organization of the written output (e.g., size, spacing, placement of writing on the page, organization of ideas), are important. In terms of more standardized tests, an assessment might include some of the following:

WIAT-II Subtests

- *Spelling.* Although not all children with dysgraphia are poor spellers, many are. Those who have grade-appropriate spelling skills will typically show poor qualitative performance on this test, such as writing with a mixture of upper- and lower-case letters or generally illegible writing.
- *Written Expression.* This subtest assesses a child's ability to write sentences and a paragraph given an extended time limit.

Woodcock–Johnson Tests of Achievement

Some of the most pertinent subtests include:

- *Spelling.*
- *Writing Fluency.* This subtest is a timed test that requires a child, in seven minutes, to formulate as many short sentences as she

can from groups of words and pictures presented in such a way as to stimulate sentence production.

- *Dictation.* This test asks the child to write dictated information, such as spelling words or correctly punctuating a sentence.

Tests of written expression, such as:

- *Rey–Osterrieth Complex Figure Test.* (See Chapter Four for more information)
- *Developmental Test of Visual–Motor Integration (VMI).* (See Chapter Four for more information)
- *Test of Written Language (TOWL).* On this test the child is asked to write a story about a picture in fifteen minutes. The story is scored according to how well it's constructed and whether proper spelling, punctuation, grammar, and vocabulary are used.

Q: My child is in kindergarten and having problems with drawing and writing. If disorder of written expression can't be diagnosed until first or second grade, is there anything I can do now to help him?

A: If you're interested in having your child evaluated at this age, we'd recommend starting with an occupational therapy evaluation. The first step would be to talk with your child's teacher as to whether she feels an evaluation is a good idea. If she does, it might be best to have the school's occupational therapist complete the evaluation. If your child's teacher feels there is no cause for concern, you still have a few options. You can request that the school's occupational therapist complete an evaluation (see Chapter Two for how to do this), or you could decide to have your child evaluated in a private occupational therapy clinic. However, if your child seems to be having difficulties in more than just writing (such as problems with prereading skills, socializing with other children, or hyperactivity), you'll want to talk with your child's teacher as to whether a more comprehensive evaluation is needed at this time.

Preparing for an Evaluation of Disorder of Written Expression

Similar to what we said earlier in the chapter, when we discussed preparing for a math disorder evaluation, if you suspect your child has problems with written expression, you'll want to have him evaluated by a professional such as a licensed psychologist. Because written expression factors into many of the tests (even those that don't specifically test writing), your child may find the evaluation tiring. However, the child generally won't be asked to write more than he would in a traditional classroom setting, as writing is an important component of many school programs today. Most examiners will keep the testing upbeat by interspersing written tests with those that are not written and by taking frequent breaks.

The Testing's Completed: Now What Do I Do?

Testing can be quite useful in determining what particular types of treatments will be most helpful for an individual child. (See the sidebar "Things to Keep in Mind after You Receive the Report" in Chapter Six.) Testing can, for example, determine whether the child's problems are due to problems with spatial organization or whether the difficulties are so severe that occupational therapy would be indicated. Testing can pinpoint other factors, such as inattention, that may be contributing to a child's difficulties.

Treatment

Treatment for disorder of written expression generally falls into one of four areas: reducing the amount of written work, modifying the assignments to meet the child's individual needs, remediating the problem by providing therapy or instruction for improving handwriting, or providing special education services or tutoring in organizing and generating ideas. Some specific approaches that are often recommended include the following:

- Allow more time for written tasks and allow students to begin projects or assignments early.
- Provide assistance with note taking, either in the form of a scribe or by providing an outline or teacher-made notes.
- Teach the child organizational aspects of writing that break the writing process into manageable stages, such as brainstorming a topic, writing a topic sentence, writing first drafts, editing, proofreading, and so forth.

What Should I Tell My Child about the Diagnosis?

Kids who have had difficulty with math or handwriting typically are well aware of their problems. In many ways it's a relief for them to know that the problems are due to a learning disability and not to their being "stupid" or "lazy." As we indicated in the chapter on dyslexia, when you tell your child in age-appropriate language about his learning disability, you're confirming what the child has already known. Let your child know that everyone has strengths and weaknesses and that testing showed, for example, that his weaknesses are in the area of written expression. Explain that you and his teacher are going to help make writing (or math) easier. Reinforce the idea that a learning disability doesn't mean that he isn't smart but that certain areas of learning are more challenging. If either you or your spouse had a learning disability as a child, talk to him about how it affected you. Finally, provide your child with resources about his disability. The books listed at the end of this chapter can help get you started. Your child's school psychologist or guidance counselor can also be an important resource.

- Encourage the child to type, to use spell checkers, and to have someone else proofread his work.
- Let the child choose between cursive or printing.
- Reduce the copying elements of assignments and tests and stress quality over quantity in written assignments.
- Offer alternatives to writing, such as an oral book report or a visual project.
- Provide the child with occupational therapy.
- Teach alternative handwriting methods such as "Handwriting without Tears" (see the resource list in this chapter).

Resources

Books for Parents

Cicci, R. (1995). *What's wrong with me?: Learning disabilities at home and at school*. Toronto, Canada: York Press.—Discusses some of the more common learning disabilities and offers suggestions on treatment.

Fisher, G., & Cummings, R. (1995). *When your child has LD (learning differences):*

A survival guide for parents. Minneapolis, MN: Free Spirit.—Describes how learning differences can affect a child's self-esteem, school performance, and future.

Olsen, J. (2001). *Handwriting without tears*. (Available from the author, 8001 MacArthur Boulevard, Cabin John, MD 20818; *www.hwtears.com*)

Richards, R. G. (1998). *Dysgraphia: The writing dilemma*. Riverside, CA: RET Center Press.—Describes ways of identifying students with dysgraphia, outlines the stages of writing, and lists specific helps for students with dysgraphia.

Books for Children

Abeel, S. (1997). *Reach for the moon*. Minneapolis, MN: Pfeifer-Hamilton.—The story of Samantha, a thirteen-year-old girl with a math disability. Samantha tells about her difficulties in middle school through poems and stories.

Kent, D., & Quinlan, K. (1996). *Extraordinary people with disabilities*. Minneapolis, MN: Children's Press.—Profiles fifty famous men and women, such as Thomas Edison, Harriet Tubman, and Tom Cruise, who have lived with a variety of disabilities.

Web Sites

www.LDonline.org—This Web site includes a wealth of information for children with various types of learning disabilities.

Eleven

Children at the Extremes: Mental Retardation and Giftedness

You may be wondering why we've chosen to include these two very different groups of individuals in one chapter. The first reason is that, by definition, children in each of these groups fall far outside the normal curve on measures of intelligence, so IQ testing figures in strongly for both groups. Second, some of the problems presented in each of these groups of children parallel one another.

About 1 to 3 percent of the school-age population could be classified as mentally retarded. According to the 1992 definition of the American Association on Mental Retardation, mental retardation refers to "substantial limitations in present functioning" characterized by "significantly subaverage intellectual functioning, existing concurrently with related limitations in two or more of the following applicable adaptive skills areas: communication, self-care, home living, social skills, community use, self-direction, health and safety, functional academics, leisure and work."

Mental retardation is considered a childhood disorder that manifests before the age of eighteen years. As you can see from the definition, to be classified as mentally retarded, a child must have below-average intellec-

Mental retardation is intellectual functioning that is significantly below average and that also occurs with related limitations in two or more adaptive skills—skills that are needed to adapt to one's living environment.

tual functioning, as well as problems with adaptive skills. Measuring intellectual functioning is fairly straightforward because standard IQ tests are typically given. Measuring adaptive functioning can be trickier, although there are some standardized measurements, which we describe below.

About 3 to 5 percent of children could be considered gifted and talented. Gifted children can be gifted in a number of areas, including intelligence, creative or artistic abilities, specific academic abilities (e.g., gifted at math), or leadership skills. Although intellectual abilities represent only one type of exceptionality, it would be rare to classify a child as gifted without administering an IQ test. Gifted children have often been stereotyped as unsociable "nerds," but research suggests that most gifted children do not fit that stereotype. However, being a gifted student is not a guarantee of success in school. For example, the verbal precocity of a gifted child (which might lead a child to dominate class discussions) can be interpreted by some teachers as disruptive or inappropriate. Peers can sometimes be less than supportive of a child whose math skills are years ahead of his class's. We sometimes see children who were never identified as intellectually gifted at an early age but who by adolescence are feeling depressed and bored with school. They've been mislabeled as "oppositional" or "lazy" because they've failed to complete assignments that they see as "dumb" or "mindless." Then there is the possibility that a child can have both above-average intelligence and another problem, such as ADHD. This presents an interesting challenge to the classroom teacher, who must keep a hyperactive, information-hungry child motivated in the classroom. Testing can be very useful in identifying the cause of these types of problem behaviors.

Mental Retardation

Robert was a friendly seventeen-year-old who was referred for testing to help plan for his future as he approached young adulthood. Robert was born with Down syndrome, a chromosomal abnormality that typically results in mental retardation, distinct physical features, and speech problems. Robert had been tested numerous times in the past, and it was determined that he had moderate mental retardation. He had been educated in the public schools and had done quite well. Robert was able to read the newspaper (especially his beloved sports page), tell time, and use money correctly. He was learning important job skills and was employed as a busboy and dishwasher at a local restaurant through his school's job placement program.

Down syndrome is a disorder caused by an extra chromosome on the twenty-first pair. It causes mental retardation that typically falls in the mild to moderate range.

There was some concern, however, about where Robert should go from here: Should he continue to receive academic instruction, or should vocational skills be emphasized in his program? Robert's parents also needed documentation that indicated he met criteria for a disability so that he would be eligible for Social Security benefits in the future.

Robert was tested using the Stanford–Binet Intelligence Scale. His Full Scale IQ was measured at 49. On tests of adaptive functioning, Robert was noted to be able to dress himself, take care of all his self-help needs, and travel independently to and from work. However, he was also noted to have significant deficits in other adaptive skills. For example, although he was able to get back and forth to work, he was not able to find his way to other places in his town independently. Academically, although his reading skills were at the fourth-grade level, his math skills were that of an early second grader. Similarly, although Robert could use a microwave oven without any difficulty, he did not have sufficient skills to use a gas oven. These types of difficulties, when combined with his performance on an IQ test, documented the fact that Robert met criteria for moderate mental retardation.

Parents often torment themselves with speculation about how their child came to be mentally retarded. The causes of mental retardation in fact are quite numerous and include such things as genetic disorders, chromosomal abnormalities, fetal alcohol syndrome, lead poisoning, and other environmental toxins. For many children, particularly those with mild retardation, the cause of the difficulties will remain unknown. If your child is mentally retarded or if you suspect he is, you and your child are best served by your focusing on how to help the child make the most of his abilities.

As in Robert's case, one of the more common chromosomal abnormalities is Down syndrome. Other genetic factors include fragile X syndrome (a condition in which the bottom of the X chromosome is pinched off), phenylketonuria (also known as PKU, a metabolic genetic disorder caused by the body's inability to convert a common dietary substance, phenylaline, to tyrosine, which can result in abnormal brain development), and Tay–Sachs disease (an inherited condition that results in brain damage and eventual death).

Infections in the mother during pregnancy, such as rubella, syphilis, or herpes simplex, are also possible risk factors for retardation. Infections in the child that can result in mental retardation include meningitis, encephalitis, or pediatric AIDS.

Finally, environmental hazards—such as a blow to a child's head, fetal alcohol syndrome, maternal drug use during pregnancy, lead poisoning, radiation to the unborn fetus, improper nutrition during pregnancy, extreme prematurity, and a loss of oxygen during pregnancy or delivery (known as anoxia)—are all risk factors for mental retardation. For more information on these and other disorders, check the resources list at the end of this chapter.

Diagnosing Mental Retardation

As Robert's case illustrates, tests of intelligence and adaptive functioning are necessary to confirm a diagnosis of mental retardation. Tests of intelligence are completed with the child, whereas tests of adaptive functioning are typically checklists completed by a person who knows the child well, such as a parent, teacher, social worker, psychologist, or mental health worker.

In most cases (perhaps as many as 90 percent) the cause of mental retardation is unknown. Regardless, cognitive, psychological, and/or neuropsychological testing is important as a descriptive measure of a child's current functioning and can help to determine program needs and future goals.

What the Evaluation Should Include

Other tests are often used as well, particularly behavioral rating scales, tests of language, and tests of academic ability. As a result, a thorough evaluation will include:

- An interview with the parents that includes information about the child's developmental, family, medical, and school history
- An intelligence test (see Chapter Four for more information on these) such as the

- ◦ Stanford–Binet
- ◦ Wechsler Intelligence Scale for Children (WISC-IV) or Wechsler Adult Intelligence Scale (WAIS-III)
- Tests of adaptive behavior such as the
  - ◦ *American Association on Mental Deficiency (AAMD) Adaptive Behavior Scales*, which are behavior rating scales that can be used with mentally retarded or developmentally disabled individuals, ages three to sixty-nine years, who are institutionalized
  - ◦ *Vineland Adaptive Behavior Scales*, which assess social competence in individuals ages birth through nineteen years. They measure the ability to perform daily activities and the ability to be socially sufficient.
  - ◦ *Adaptive Behavior Inventory for Children*, which measures behavior in the home, neighborhood, and community. Items ask about the child's family life, ability to function in school, social relationships, leisure activities, and ability to perform household chores.

Other tests, although not necessary to make a diagnosis of mental retardation, might include:

- Tests of language ability, such as the Peabody Picture Vocabulary Test (PPVT-III), the Expressive Vocabulary Test (EVT), or the Boston Naming Test (see Chapter Four for more information)
- Tests of executive functions to determine whether there are significant attention difficulties (see Chapter Seven for more information)
- Tests of academic functioning, such as math and reading achievement tests

How Intelligence Tests Are Used to Diagnose Mental Retardation

Take another look at the normal bell-shaped curve you first saw in Chapter Five. Children with mental retardation have IQ scores that fall in the shaded area shown on the curve. The vast majority (around 85 to 90 percent) of the mentally retarded have scores that fall in the range of 50 to 70 on IQ tests. These children are classified as having mild mental retardation. Although their development is nearly always slower than average, their retardation often isn't identified until they reach school, when their difficulties become more apparent. Those with moderate mental retardation—IQ scores ranging from 35 to 40 to 50 to 55—typically are slow to develop language and motor skills and as a result are often placed in early intervention programs, preschool programs for developmentally delayed youngsters. Moderately retarded individuals can learn academic skills (although at a slower rate than the nondisabled) and are capable of learning occupational and social skills. They can hold jobs, although they require moderate levels of supervision. Individuals with severe or profound mental retardation have very limited abilities. They often have little or no speech, poor motor control, and may need twenty-four-hour care. However, they are capable of learning self-help skills such as dressing and eating and sometimes can learn to do simple jobs under close supervision.

Mild mental retardation: IQ scores ranging from 50–55 to around 70

Moderate mental retardation: IQ scores ranging from 35–40 to 50–55

Severe mental retardation: IQ scores ranging from 20–25 to 35–40

Profound mental retardation: IQ scores below 20 or 25

Preparing for an Evaluation for Mental Retardation

It's difficult to predict how long an evaluation for mental retardation will take, because it depends on the child's attention span and the number of tests completed. It will typically take one to two hours to complete an IQ test. If other tests are completed as well, the testing could

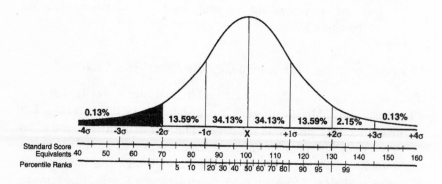

Normal curve indicating distribution of IQ scores for children with mental retardation.

Q: My foster child's IQ was measured at 60, which would place him in the mild mentally retarded range, yet his adaptive functioning is normal for his age. In fact, he took care of himself from an early age, as he came from an abusive home and was neglected for much of his life. Does this IQ score mean he's retarded?

A: No, your foster child would not be considered retarded for a couple of reasons. First, if he is functioning at age level in his ability to adapt to his environment, he would not meet the criteria for mental retardation. Second, if he was abused or neglected for much of his life, it is quite possible that his IQ score can be attributed to a lack of stimulation in his environment. Hopefully, with an enriched, loving environment and the right educational interventions, he may perform better on future measures of intelligence.

---

take considerably longer. It's generally a good idea to do the testing over a few shorter time periods. This type of testing is very often completed within the school setting. However, sometimes schools refer a child to an outside evaluator so that they can get an independent measure of functioning. This can be particularly true for children with mental retardation, who can be difficult to test because of a lack of language skills or behavior problems. Parents sometimes seek an outside evaluation so they can get a second opinion. This type of independent evaluation is very often covered by insurance because the child typically has a medical diagnosis that requires a need for testing.

In terms of preparing your child for the testing, how you do so depends on her level of understanding. If your child has good language comprehension, let him know that he'll need to see a doctor who will be asking him to do things such as name pictures, put puzzles together, and draw. If your child's ability to comprehend is limited, prepare her in the way you think is best. It is generally not a good idea to wait until you walk through the doctor's office door to tell her she is being tested. If your child is being tested in school, she will generally think the testing is just part of the normal things she is expected to do at school, and as a result little explanation is typically provided.

In general, we've found that it's best to keep things simple and clear. Overexplaining the purpose of the testing is not productive; however, not explaining the testing to a child with mental retardation is unfair and may compromise the results if the child becomes angry that he didn't know. Most school-age children with mental retardation are quite used to seeing many different types of professionals (speech/language therapists, occupational therapists, etc.) in the course of the normal school day, so they often don't experience the testing as outside of their normal realm of experience, even if the testing is completed outside the school setting.

The Testing's Completed: Now What Do I Do?

In most cases, test results can be extremely helpful in guiding your child's mental health care team in devising future programs. (See the sidebar "Things to Keep in Mind after You Receive the Report" in Chapter Six.) For example, testing provides information about a child's progress in academic subjects such as reading and math. It provides information about a child's learning strengths and weaknesses so that treatment can be tailored to build on his strengths and treat his weaknesses. It can determine whether a child needs training in self-help skills (eating, dressing, grooming), home management skills (cleaning, laundry, cooking), consumer skills (use of money, shopping), or mobility skills (the ability to use public transportation).

Cindy, a fourteen-year-old with mild mental retardation as a result of oxygen loss during the birth process, was a very friendly, warm young adolescent with extremely good social and language skills. However, when tested, it was revealed that Cindy could read few words. Her inability to read had been attributed to her mental retardation; however, testing indicated she was quite capable of reading—she just had never been taught. Unfortunately, her lack of reading skills resulted in Cindy's not being able to use public transportation, as she couldn't read the bus destinations. Testing indicated that she had the cognitive skills to be able to use public transportation but was lacking the literacy skills. As a result, it was recommended that Cindy get intense support in literacy skills. Within a year, Cindy was able to read at an early-second-grade level. Testing continued to be useful in Cindy's case because it provided a measure of her reading improvement over the course of her treatment.

Treatment

As you might expect, there is a wide range of treatment options for children with mental retardation, with treatment dependent on the severity and nature of the retardation. Most children with mental retardation need some sort of special education services. Mildly mentally retarded

What Should I Tell My Child about the Diagnosis?

This is a difficult question to answer because it depends greatly on your child's level of understanding. Our recommendation would be to provide the child with as much information about her disability as she is able to understand. For instance, many individuals with Down syndrome are quite aware of their condition and what mental retardation means. In contrast, children with severe or profound mental retardation would benefit very little from information about their disorder. There is almost a limitless list of resources to help you with this dilemma. We've listed a few at the end of the chapter to help get you started.

children are most often educated within the normal school environment, either in special self-contained classes, through mainstreaming (being placed in classes with nonretarded peers), or in some combination of the two. Often, their early school years are spent learning academic subjects, and later school years focus more on vocational training. At the other end of the spectrum, education for severely and profoundly retarded children typically focuses more on survival skills, self-help, and communication skills. Treatment often focuses on reducing inappropriate behaviors such as rocking or tantrums. Education for these children often occurs in special schools or residential treatment centers.

Regardless of the age of your child, if he has been found to be retarded or is at risk for retardation (e.g., is an infant with Down syndrome, PKU, extreme prematurity, etc.), he is entitled to a free public education from the age of three to twenty-one. Your child is also entitled to education in the "least restrictive environment," the environment that allows him to develop to his potential with the fewest barriers while maintaining sufficient support. If your child is younger than age three, find out if your school district offers an early intervention program, as prevention of mental retardation depends on early identification and treatment.

Giftedness

Sue's mother, Lisa, was quite concerned. Lisa volunteered as a teacher's helper in Sue's kindergarten class every week, and what she'd observed worried her. Sue didn't seem to be interested in many of the things the other children liked. Sue was an avid reader who read at the fourth-grade level. Lisa had difficulty finding books that challenged Sue's ability to read yet were age-appropriate in content. Many of the children in Sue's class were just beginning to learn letter–sound correspondences, while Sue was reading chapter books. Although Sue didn't have any difficulty making friends outside of school, within the school environment she often looked as if she felt left out. When she was asked to solve a math problem in a group of students, Sue immediately knew the answer. She realized that if she said the answer out loud, the teacher would reprimand her; however, she felt bored and frustrated waiting for her friends to find out how to solve the problems. A few parents complained that it wasn't fair that Sue got special attention from the teacher just because she already knew how to read. They wanted special attention for their children, too. Lisa felt there must be something wrong with her child. Why else would she be causing such trouble?

Lisa took Sue to a psychologist, who administered an intelligence test and completed a few tests of emotional functioning and some behavioral rating scales. The results indicated that Sue was quite bright. Her Full Scale IQ on the Wechsler Preschool and Primary Scale of Intelligence (WPPSI) was 145—three standard deviations above the average range. The tests of emotional functioning indicated that Sue didn't have any significant difficulties but often felt lonely. Despite her high intelligence, she didn't feel smart. Behavioral rating scales completed by her parents and teacher indicated she had no problem areas. In sum, Sue's intelligence was far superior to that of her peers, which was leading to some problems within the classroom setting. This is not uncommon, as a child who achieves far above her peers is subject to criticism or social isolation not only from other children but also from other students' parents as well. Once the testing was completed and the results discussed with her parents, they decided that a private school for the gifted would be the best placement for her.

Diagnosing Giftedness

The special needs of the gifted child have traditionally received much less attention than the other disorders we've discussed in this book. In part, this is because giftedness is not a "disorder" in need of treatment but something to be fostered. However, gifted students are often referred for testing because something isn't fitting for them. In Sue's case, her mother had a gut feeling that her child wasn't like other children. In other cases, gifted children may be so far ahead of their age-mates that they already know much of the curriculum before it is even taught. Their boredom sometimes results in low achievement and grades. In contrast, gifted students can be quite perfectionistic and may define success as not just getting 100 on a test but getting a 100 plus all the extra credit points. Their high standards can lead to a fear of failure and, at worst, feelings of low self-esteem and depression.

By definition, people who are gifted have above-average intelligence and/or superior talent for something, such as music, art, or math. Most public school programs for the gifted select children who have superior intellectual skills and academic aptitude. Children with a superior talent for something (arts, drama, dance) aren't typically provided with services within the school setting but instead take classes in their ability. There are a few exceptions to this, as some school districts do have special schools for the sciences or for the performing or visual arts, such as seen in the movie *Fame*.

What the Testing Evaluation Should Include

There are no tests to identify children with a superior talent in music or the arts, because talent is somewhat subjective. However, as you've probably guessed, a number of tests can identify children with superior intelligence. See Chapter Four for more information on intelligence testing, which could include:

- Wechsler Preschool and Primary Scale of Intelligence (WPPSI)
- Wechsler Intelligence Scale for Children (WISC)
- Wechsler Adult Intelligence Scale (WAIS)
- Stanford–Binet Intelligence Scales

Other tests can also be used, depending on what difficulties or attributes the child may have. For example, we've tested many children who have superior intelligence and ADHD, dyslexia, and/or handwriting problems. If that's the case, the evaluation will include test batteries described in previous chapters. Sometimes, as in Sue's case, it's not initially clear that the child's problems are due to giftedness. In those cases, tests of emotional functioning (e.g., projective tests, behavioral rating scales, or self-report measures; see Chapter Four) may be given.

Preparing for an Evaluation for Giftedness

Be frank with your child as to why you're seeking testing. Let her know that you're interested in getting an idea of how she learns best. If you are seeking testing because you have some concerns (such as that you suspect your child is not achieving at her potential), let her know that you want to get ideas on how to make her school experience successful. Sometimes parents seek evaluations in the hopes of getting their child into a private school or enrichment program. If that's the case, don't put any undue pressure on your child, such as saying "You have to ace this test or you won't get into the XXX School!"

Most gifted kids love the testing process, because intelligence tests are generally fun for them. If they are completing just an intelligence test and a few other measures, the testing will usually take one to two hours. This type of testing is *never* covered by insurance. You can expect to pay $300 to $500 or more for this simple evaluation and much more if you have additional concerns or interests.

How Intelligence Tests Are Used to Determine Whether a Child Is Gifted

Here again is the normal bell-shaped curve we've shown earlier in this chapter. The shaded area includes a little over 2 percent of the population, the top 2 percent of the population with IQs above 130. This is an arguable cutoff for giftedness, because some people would define giftedness more broadly—as being in the top 20 percent of the popula-

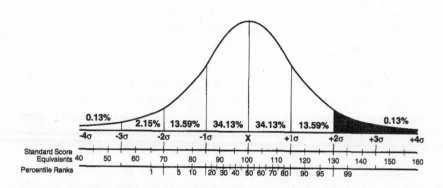

Normal curve indicating distribution of IQ scores for gifted children.

Q: If my child has a high IQ, is she entitled to special services?

A: No. Giftedness is not a disability in any usual sense, and it is not defined in the IDEA (Individuals with Disabilities Education Act; see Chapter Two for more information). Although many school districts provide programs for the gifted, many do not. Federal law encourages school districts to provide services for gifted children. Sadly, however, in times of budget shortfalls, gifted education is often seen as an unnecessary luxury.

tion—whereas others would define it less broadly—as being in the top 1 percent of the population.

The Testing's Completed: Now What Do I Do?

Although schools are not required to provide special services for gifted children, many do, and most programs fall into two categories: enrichment experiences (giving students additional learning experiences without moving them up a grade) and acceleration (placing gifted students in grade levels ahead of their peers). Enrichment services can occur within the classroom or outside the classroom, as in a resource-room setting. Sometimes schools will provide gifted students with mentors outside the school environment. For example, a gifted math student might be mentored by a member of the community who has special skills in this area (e.g., a chemist, engineer, or astrophysicist). Some school districts offer special schools for gifted and talented students. These school districts are typically located in large metropolitan areas. There are also many good private school choices for gifted children.

Because there's no federal definition of gifted and talented, each state has its own criteria for identifying students and providing services. If you think your child might be gifted, you may want to start by talking to your child's teacher or principal to discuss options for testing your child and possibilities for specialized programming. Even if your school doesn't provide services, testing can be helpful. If testing indicates your child is gifted, you can enroll him in after-school programs. Most metropolitan areas have programs that are offered through museums, community education centers, or universities. For example, if your child was tested and it was determined she was quite gifted on

What Do I Tell My Child about the Diagnosis?

Let your child know that the test results showed that he is very smart and that he'll often learn at a quicker pace than other children his age. If you sought an evaluation for your child because something wasn't going well, use the results to reinforce the child's strengths. As we indicated earlier, some gifted children don't feel as though they're very smart. However, if the testing also was useful in determining your child's areas of weakness (and why he's having trouble), share that with him as well in age-appropriate language. It's also important to let your child know that being smart doesn't necessarily mean that he'll be advanced in all areas. Everyone has areas of relative difficulty, and so he shouldn't expect everything to be easy for him. Most important, let your child know that being different from other children doesn't necessarily mean he is *better* than other children, as arrogance or bragging can contribute to social problems.

most of the tests of verbal ability, you might want to enroll her in a writing class. We've listed a number of resources at the end of the chapter that can get you started. Some of the Web sites we've listed have information regarding local chapters or services.

Resources on Mental Retardation

Books for Parents

Bogdan R., & Taylor, S. (1994). *The social meaning of mental retardation: Two life stories* (Special Education, No. 15). New York: Teachers' College Press.

Cunningham, C. (1996). *Understanding Down syndrome: An introduction for parents.* Cambridge, MA: Brookline Books.

Stray-Gunderson, K. (Ed.). (1995). *Babies with Down syndrome: A new parents guide* (The Special Needs Collection). Bethesda, MD: Woodbine House.

Books for Kids

Becker, S. (1991). *Buddy's shadow.* Hollidaysburg, PA: Jason and Nordic.—A five-year-old boy with Down's Syndrome buys a puppy.

Berkus, C. W. (1992). *Charlie's chuckle.* Woodbine House.—About a seven-year-old boy with Down syndrome.

Butler, G. (1998). *The Hangashore*. Toronto, Canada: Tundra Books.—A man with Down syndrome displays courage and kindness.

Carter, A. R. (1997). *Big brother Dustin*. Morton Grove, IL: Whitman.—A young boy with Down syndrome learns that his parents are going to have a baby.

Glatzer, J. (2002). *Taking Down syndrome to school*. Plainview, NY: JayJo Books.

Holcomb, N. (1987). *How about a hug?* Hollidaysburg, PA: Jason and Nordic.— The story of a young girl with Down's syndrome that details a typical day in her life.

Rickert, J. E. (2000). *Russ and the almost perfect day*. Bethesda, MD: Woodbine House.

Rickert, J. E. (1999). *Russ and the apple tree surprise*. Bethesda, MD: Woodbine House.

Rickert, J. E. (2000). *Russ and the fire house*. Bethesda, MD: Woodbine House.

Stuve-Bodeen, S. (1998). *We'll paint the octopus red*. Bethesda, MD: Woodbine House.—The story of a little girl who has a new baby brother with Down syndrome.

Thompson, M. (1992). *My brother, Matthew*. Bethesda, MD: Woodbine House.—A boy describes life with a younger brother who has a mental disability.

Wright, B. R. (1990). *My sister is different*. Barrington, IL: Steck-Vaughn.—What it's like to have an older sister with mental retardation.

Organizations/Web Sites

American Association on Mental Retardation (AAMR)
444 North Capital Street, NW
Suite 846
Washington, DC 20001-1512
800-424-3688
www.aamr.org
—An organization of professionals working in the field of mental retardation.

ARC of the United States
1010 Wayne Avenue, Suite 650
Silver Spring, MD 20910
301-565-3842
info@thearc.org
www.thearc.org
—Formerly the Association for Retarded Citizens, the ARC is a volunteer organization committed to the welfare of children and adults with mental retardation and their families.

Council for Exceptional Children
1110 North Glebe Road
Suite 300
Arlington, VA 22201-5704
1-888-CEC-SPED
www.cec.sped.org

People First International
P.O. Box 12642
Salem, OR 97309
503-362-0336
   —A self-advocacy organization of people with mental retardation or other developmental disabilities who meet in local chapters.

President's Committee on Mental Retardation
www.ncor.org/pcmr.htm
   —Provides publications promoting the quality of life and inclusion of people with disabilities.

Resources on Giftedness

Books for Parents

Halstead, J. W. (1995). *Some of my best friends are books: Guiding gifted readers from preschool to high school*. Scottsdale, AZ: Great Potential.

Kerr, B. A. (1997). *Smart girls: A new psychology of girls, women, and giftedness* (rev. ed.). Scottsdale, AZ: Great Potential.

Kerr, B. A., Cohn, S., Webb, J. T., & Andersen, T. (2001). *Smart boys: Talent, manhood, and the search for meaning*. Scottsdale, AZ: Great Potential.

Neihart, M., Reis, S. M., Robinson, N. M., & Moon, S. M. (Eds.). (2001). *The social and emotional development of gifted children: What do we know?* Waco, TX: Prufrock.—Covers topics of interest to parents and teachers and includes chapters on peer pressure and social acceptance, delinquency, and underachievement, among others. The book also reviews the research literature with regard to gifted students.

Helping gifted children soar: A practical guide for parents and teachers. Scottsdale, AZ: Great Potential.

Books for Kids

Galbraith, J., Espeland, P., & Molnar, A. (1998). *The gifted kids' survival guide for ages 10 & under*. Minneapolis, MN: Free Spirit.—A book written for gifted children, which answers questions such as why they think and act the way they do, what IQs really mean, and how to deal with their—and others'—high expectations.

Organizations/Web Sites

American Association for Gifted Children at Duke University
Box 90270
Durham, NC 27708
www.aagc.org

ERIC Clearinghouse on Disabilities and Gifted Education
1110 North Glebe Road
Arlington, VA 22201-5704
800-328-0272
ericec.org

Twelve

Depression, Anxiety, and Other Psychological Concerns

Millions of kids each year are evaluated for psychiatric concerns such as depression and anxiety. Although psychological testing, or testing that provides information about your child's emotional and behavioral functioning, is not always essential for diagnosing problems such as depression, it is frequently quite helpful in shedding light on the underlying contributing factors. Psychological testing can also provide information about the severity of the condition, as well as opportunities for treatment. Often people, kids and adults alike, are not entirely aware of what might be driving their anxiety or sadness. Certain tests called *projective tests* are thought to provide a window into a person's inner world, tapping into conflicts, wishes, and the like that the person may not be able or ready to access directly on his own. These tests, in combination with a thorough history, self-report measures, parent-report measures, clinical interview, and observation, typically provide useful information about your child that otherwise might not be obtained through a basic psychiatric evaluation.

> Because fourteen-year-old Nicole had become irritable and withdrawn over the past few months of high school, her mother was concerned that she might be depressed. Nicole's mother contacted an area child psychologist who recommended a full neuropsychological and psychological evaluation. Nicole's parents were glad that they had been given a direction to go in to help their daughter, but what would testing re-

ally do for her? How would it help them figure out why she was so moody?

Depression

Many children like Nicole develop signs of possible mood disorders, such as depression. Depression is the most common of the mood disorders and affects about 2 to 5 percent of all school-age children and adolescents; generally, the older the child, the higher her risk of becoming depressed. Until adolescence, depression is as common in boys as it is in girls; by about age thirteen and up, however, roughly 65 percent of the cases are girls. Children and adults who are depressed tend to show at least five of the following symptoms for at least two weeks:

Signs of Depression

1. Depressed mood most of the day, nearly every day; in kids, often appears as increased irritability or a "shorter fuse"
2. A loss of interest in many or most things, such as school, friends, activities
3. Weight gain or loss of about 5 percent of the child's original body weight or a noticeable increase or decrease in appetite
4. A noticeable increase or decrease in sleep
5. An increase in restlessness or fidgety behavior *or* a decrease in the child's usual level of activity
6. Feeling tired or having low energy almost every day
7. Feelings of worthlessness, guilt, and/or general low self-confidence
8. A decrease in the child's ability to concentrate and/or to make decisions nearly every day
9. Recurrent thoughts of death and/or of harming or killing oneself; this may include suicidal statements or attempts

It's important to know that depression and other mood disorders such as bipolar disorder tend to run in families. Children with at least one parent who has experienced depression have at least a one and a half to three times greater risk of also becoming depressed. It can be tough, however, to figure out whether your child is actually depressed or just going through "growing pains" or "a phase." Nicole, for example, recently started menstruating, began going to a new school, and started getting a lot more homework. Her father thought she was simply reacting to normal life stressors and would eventually improve. After a few months, however, she seemed worse rather than better, and her parents followed through with the recommended testing evaluation.

A psychological testing evaluation for depression is often helpful in ways that a general diagnostic evaluation with a pediatrician or mental health professional is not. Self-report tests, such as the Children's Depression Inventory (CDI) and the Culture Free Self-Esteem Inventory (SEI), and parent observation questionnaires, such as the Child Behavior Checklist (CBCL) and the Behavioral Assessment System fir Children (BASC), help determine the presence and severity of the child's depression. They can provide the clinician who will be treating the depression with information about which symptoms are most prominent and what beliefs the child holds that seem to be fueling her low self-esteem. Projective testing, which includes measures such as the Rorschach or the Children's Apperception Test (CAT), gives the evaluator the opportunity to understand what may be driving the depression for the child or adolescent, particularly when she might be having difficulty understanding it herself. Sometimes a child or teenager will be quite guarded or unwilling to discuss her feelings. Here, too, projective testing can be particularly useful, as the tests tend to elicit thoughts and feelings that have been avoided or suppressed.

Anxiety

Anxiety, which is a general term for a variety of specific disorders such as separation anxiety, panic disorder, social anxiety, obsessive-compulsive disorder, posttraumatic stress disorder, and generalized anxiety disorder, is fairly common in children. It is estimated that thousands of school-age children have one type of anxiety disorder or another, and, like depression, anxiety tends to run in families. Although the labels may differ, the one uniting feature of all anxiety disorders is frequent excessive worrying or nervousness. Anxious kids tend to show a level of fearfulness beyond what would be considered typical of their developmental stage; for example, it is common for preschoolers to be afraid of monsters under their beds but not to the extent that they cannot go to sleep every night or refuse to leave their parents' sides.

It's pretty easy to spot the anxious kids who are able to tell about their fears or who behave in ways that show they feel worried—they may become tense, tearful, and clinging when they have to confront a situation that they fear. However, a good portion of anxious children appear far more angry than worried and engage in frequent, intense tantrums or anger attacks triggered by feelings of anxiety. This behavior can be more difficult to understand as being anxiety based. It's in these cases that psychological testing is often helpful in figuring out what is going on for the child.

Q: Our ten-year-old daughter has always been a little anxious, but this year she's started to be afraid of going to school. It began with unexplained stomachaches and other such "illnesses" that disappeared about an hour after I picked her up from school. Now she cries each morning, saying that she can't go to school, and it's getting almost impossible to get her out the door. What's wrong?

A: It sounds as though your daughter may have school phobia, a form of social phobia that affects children and teenagers who usually have some history of anxiety symptoms. It's particularly important for children with this type of anxiety disorder to undergo a combination of neuropsychological and psychological testing, however, because there is a good chance that something has made school a place they want to escape or avoid. This may be the social stress or level of stimulation that school imposes, but often it's a learning problem that hasn't been addressed. Even if the testing evaluation tells you what has been contributing to your daughter's school avoidance, it's likely that she would benefit from cognitive-behavioral therapy that targets her anxiety, as she may be prone to these symptoms whenever she experiences stress. With the right support and intervention, school may become tolerable or even enjoyable for kids like your daughter as they begin to find success there. Therapy will give your daughter the tools to help her deal with anxiety and hopefully make it less debilitating for her over her lifetime.

Psychotic Disorders

Fortunately, psychotic disorders, which include schizophrenia and severe forms of depression and bipolar disorder, are rare in children.
About 1 percent of children ages five to eighteen have a psychotic disorder, and although most types improve with medication, some forms
get worse over time and are lifelong.

Psychosis is considered a severe mental disorder marked by major
negative changes in a person's reasoning skills, particularly the ability
to perceive and respond appropriately to reality. Children and adults
are rarely diagnosed with a psychotic disorder unless they show signs
of having hallucinations or delusions. A child who is hallucinating may
report seeing (visual), hearing (auditory), smelling (olfactory), and/or
feeling (tactile) things that aren't really there. A child who is experiencing delusions will report a belief or thought that is highly unrealistic or
unlikely. As you might imagine, true hallucinations and delusions are
difficult to diagnose in young children given the developmental emphasis on make-believe. It is concerning to clinicians if a child, by age
four or five, cannot distinguish reality from fantasy, however. That's
why when seven-year-old Carter was certain that he was Batman and no
longer Carter, his pediatrician became concerned. When she inter-
viewed him and learned that Carter had been hearing a voice telling
him to "kill all the bad guys" for several weeks and that he firmly be-
lieved "the real Carter is dead," he was admitted to a child psychiatric
unit for observation and eventually diagnosed with a psychotic disorder.

Unlike Carter, who was fairly obviously experiencing a break with
reality, certain children and adolescents may show signs of erroneous
thinking that may or may not be caused by a psychotic disorder. Sandra, age eleven, for example, always seemed to misinterpret others'
behavior negatively, telling her mother such things as, "Amy got the
whole school against me, and now everyone hates me, even the teachers, and I can't go back to school." Sometimes her ideas were even
more troubling, such as her conviction that her brother had tried to
poison her pet hamster.

When there is a question about whether or not a child is psychotic,
psychological testing can be instrumental in diagnosing the problem.
Particular tests, such as the Rorschach and the TAT, described in Chapter Four, seem to be uniquely sensitive to the perceptual and reasoning

impairments that are associated with a psychotic disorder. Some of Carter's responses on the Rorschach included "a headless angel on fire with lobster claws and she's trying to get me!" and "mystery blood," whereas his TAT stories were rambling and illogical, with themes of being controlled by outside forces.

Neuropsychological testing also may provide information about why a child's thinking seems odd, given that there may be a processing problem or learning disability (e.g., a nonverbal learning disorder) that is contributing to his difficulties. Because psychosis may be brought on by seizure activity or brain damage that results from injury or illness, neuropsychological testing can be instrumental in determining what specific functions and skills have been affected and may guide rehabilitation therapy.

Oppositional Defiant Disorder

Many children are brought in for testing evaluations because of "bad behavior," whether it's observed and reported by the parents, teachers, or someone else who spends a lot of time with the child. Some troubling behaviors, such as tantrums, turn out to be developmentally appropriate (exasperating though they may be), and others may prove to be symptomatic of a mental health problem such as anxiety. Psychological testing can certainly help identify the anxiety, as described previously. But sometimes behavior is the primary issue, in which case the child may be diagnosed with oppositional defiant disorder (ODD) or conduct disorder (CD).

Children diagnosed with ODD typically have extreme difficulty complying with the limits set by others and often become argumentative, angry, and even explosive in their behavior. Though a child will receive this diagnosis only after these concerns have been present for at least six months, we tend to find that they have often existed for much longer, perhaps because parents believe that behavior problems are their responsibility to handle on their own.

Conduct Disorder

Conduct disorder is less common, affecting more boys than girls, and includes behaviors such as aggression toward others, destruction of property, stealing, lying, and serious violation of rules (e.g., staying out all night; skipping school repeatedly). To receive this diagnosis, a child or teenager would have to have displayed a number of these behaviors within the previous year, with at least one behavior pattern lasting six months or more. Psychological and neuropsychological testing often yields useful information about why a child may be engaging in these behaviors, as typically there are underlying cognitive and emotional concerns that have gone unaddressed or have been misunderstood.

Q: My son Michael is now eight years old. He's been hard to discipline all his life, but now his teacher is reporting that he doesn't listen to directions, gets up from his seat during class without permission, refuses to come in from recess, and routinely talks back to her during the school day. This is not the first time we've had teachers report problems with Michael's behavior, but it's certainly the worst it's ever been. What should we do to address the problem?

A: Michael sounds very familiar to us—we see many children each year who fit this description to a T. At first glance one might think Michael has a "behavior problem" or even meets criteria for ODD, but we want to stress the importance of looking for more information: What's causing Michael to behave this way? Why is his behavior worse now than before? A good evaluation that includes neuropsychological and psychological testing will likely give some answers. For example, it's quite possible that Michael has ADHD, which would help explain his difficulty listening, "shifting gears" from one activity to another, and remaining seated. He may have an undiagnosed learning disability that is causing him great frustration and in turn is contributing to his behavior problems. He may be reacting to stress in the family or in the world around him, preoccupied with worries, and angry about feeling so insecure.

Many children with ADHD are described as harder to discipline than their peers, but Michael's behavioral challenges may warrant a separate diagnosis of ODD. For this to be the case, he'd probably have to have behaved similarly or worse at home for at least six months (though usually much longer). He would also likely be prone to angry outbursts and have major trouble accepting limits from others. We think that having him evaluated by a child psychologist who will do testing is a good place to start.

Eating Disorders and Self-Mutilation

Eating disorders and self-mutilation behaviors, the latter often referred to as "cutting," continue to be prevalent among adolescent girls. Both of these concerns warrant immediate professional attention given the potentially life-threatening nature of each of these problems. Anorexia remains the most fatal of all mental disorders, and teenagers who self-mutilate have been known to unintentionally inflict injuries serious enough to cause major damage or worse. Boys may have either of these problems but are generally considered to be at lower risk than girls. Because affected young people tend to be rather emotionally guarded or have difficulty with emotional insight, psychological testing can be a useful tool for the medical and mental health professionals working with them. The projective measures in particular may provide information about the level and sources of distress for these kids and promote their recovery by providing an understanding of their difficulties.

> **Emotional insight** is the ability to reflect on one's feelings and to understand their meaning, causes, connections, and so forth.

Seventeen-year-old Lora, who had been cutting herself for years, was found to have psychological testing results that were very consistent with sexual trauma. With this as a possible contributing factor to her distress, her therapist worked with her to eventually confront her abuse history, allowing her to find healthier ways of coping with the aftermath of this trauma.

Q: My twelve-year-old daughter has started to weigh herself several times a day and talks a lot about how fat she is, even though she's not overweight. I've noticed that she is exercising a lot more and eating a lot less; I think she's even skipping lunch at school. My friends think I should have her evaluated for an eating disorder, especially before it gets out of hand. Would testing be a part of this kind of evaluation?

A: We agree with your friends that some type of intervention must take place, because eating disorders can escalate quickly and are life threatening. It is generally recommended that you consult your pediatrician first; sometimes a heart-to-heart between doctor and patient can help, particularly if the pediatrician educates your daughter about normal, healthy weight ranges for her body type, good nutrition, bodily changes due to hormones and puberty, and long-term damage to her body that can stem from drastic dieting and overexercising.

If your pediatrician or you continue to be concerned after this initial intervention because your daughter's behavior hasn't changed for the better, you may be referred for a full psychiatric evaluation, which may eventually include psychological testing. In the case of eating disorders, testing isn't necessary for diagnosis but is often quite helpful to the therapist working with the anorexic or bulimic person. By the nature of these disorders, those affected are having trouble understanding and expressing their distress adaptively. Psychological testing can sometimes provide information about what may be underlying the symptoms (e.g., feeling conflicted about growing up), thereby giving the therapist more to work with in treatment.

Diagnosing Psychological Concerns

Because the role of testing in diagnosis can vary widely depending on the disorder suspected, it's important that you ask the referring doctor exactly what questions he hopes to get answered by having your child tested. Does he need the results of neuropsychological or psychological tests to make a firm diagnosis? If so, why? Maybe he feels he has a handle on your child's primary diagnosis but that that diagnosis can't account for some of the child's symptoms, and so he wants to look for a co-occurring disorder. Or is he confident that he can make an accurate diagnosis but needs more information about your child's abilities so as to prescribe the best possible treatment?

As a parent you'll want to make sure that, if an accurate diagnosis can be made right now, you don't postpone treatment that could return your child to normal functioning and spare him needless emotional pain while you wait for testing that will answer less urgent questions. Danny's doctor was certain that he was severely depressed, even suicidal, and that he needed psychotherapy and medication as soon as possible. He requested psychological testing to help figure out what was contributing to his depression. At first, Danny's parents wanted to wait for the results of the testing evaluation, thinking they needed to have that information before knowing whether he needed therapy and medicine. Luckily, they discussed this with Danny's doctor, who explained that testing in this case wasn't being used to diagnose the problem (depression) but to provide information about *why* he was depressed in order to guide the therapy. Asking questions, as Danny's parents did, can allow you to help your child get back on track as quickly and smoothly as possible. It can also make you a wise consumer. If your doctor is unable to explain why your child needs a lengthy list of tests, you might want to seek a second opinion before making a sizable investment of time and money.

What the Testing Evaluation Should Include

Although the specific measures will likely vary from psychologist to psychologist and place to place, it is considered essential to perform more than one psychological test as part of an assessment. The use of only one test to figure out how a person is thinking and feeling is sort of like having just one piece to a puzzle—with only that much information, how can you figure out what the picture is? At times a psychological screening may be completed first, to determine whether a follow-up full evaluation would be helpful or is necessary. With a screening, one or two measures may be used.

> A *psychological screening* is a brief assessment of your child's emotional and behavioral functioning using only a couple of tests.

If your child has been referred for a full psychological evaluation to assess her emotional and/or behavioral functioning, you should expect the professional working with you to perform most of the following tests or types of tests, in addition to a taking a thorough history and performing a clinical interview with you and your child.

Projective Tests

Though psychologists in certain parts of the country are more apt to use several projective measures than others, it's reasonable to expect your child to receive the Rorschach, or inkblot, test, as well as an apperception test such as the Children's Apperception Test (CAT), the Roberts Apperception Test for Children (RATC), or the Thematic Apperception Test (TAT). These storytelling tests, as they are sometimes called, typically provide information about how your child sees himself and others, as well as the major conflicts or issues that may be contributing to his distress. Information about his coping skills, ability to judge situations realistically, and social skills is also often gleaned from these tests' results.

Other projective tests include drawings, such as in the Draw-A-Person test, House–Tree–Person test, and Kinetic Family Drawing test. Sentence completion tests are somewhat projective in nature, as they function similar to word association tasks. On these tests kids are asked to finish a sentence that the evaluator starts for them. Sentence stems such as "My friends . . . ," "At home I . . . ," and, "In school . . ." may yield information about how your child feels about himself and the world around him.

Apperception tests are projective measures that use pictures of different scenes and situations. The child is asked to tell a story about each picture, giving his interpretation of what he sees.

Self-Report Measures

For children ages six and up, self-report measures, or tests that ask a child directly about her thoughts and feelings, have been developed. The Children's Depression Inventory, for example, consists of several grouped statements (e.g., "I feel sad all the time," "I feel sad once in a while," etc.), and the child needs to choose which one best describes her. This can be read to a younger child, or the child can complete it on her own if she is at least a first- or second-grade-level reader. The Culture Free Self-Esteem Inventory is another such measure on which the child indicates "yes" or "no" in response to a statement such as "I need more friends." This test gives the evaluator a sense of how the child feels about himself in various contexts (socially, at school, at home, physically).

For older kids and teens, measures such as the Millon Adolescent Personality Inventory (MAPI) and the MMPI-A have been developed. After the child has answered many true/false questions about herself, the responses are analyzed and clustered into many different factors, such as social satisfaction, assertiveness, depression, and the like.

Parent-Report/Teacher-Report Measures

It's important to determine how your child is seen and experienced by you and other adults in his life, such as teachers or coaches. Although you probably can't be totally objective, you know your child best, and the psychologist working with you would be leaving a very critical stone unturned if she did not involve you in the evaluation process. Likewise, teachers spend a significant amount of time with our kids and often get to observe them under very different conditions (e.g., with a large group, out on the playground without much supervision, etc.). Their input is usually very helpful in determining what's going on with your child and how to help. Measures such as the BASC (parent and teacher forms) and the CBCL (parent and teacher forms) offer a thorough list of questions about your child's social, behavioral, and emotional functioning.

Referral for Educational or Neuropsychological Testing

We can think of numerous instances in which educational and/or neuropsychological testing was able to shed important light on the emotional or behavioral problems that kids were having. It will be important for the clinician working with your child to consider the role your child's wiring and cognitive style plays in how he copes with the world around him. Hidden learning disabilities, too, frequently lurk behind anxiety and depression in kids, particularly as children spend the majority of their days in an academic setting in which they are reminded of their "inadequacies." We encourage you to ask the evaluator about the need for further testing, as it could be overlooked otherwise.

Preparing for a Psychological Evaluation

Testing evaluations for psychological concerns usually take from one to three hours of testing, with needed breaks. You as the parent will need to take part in the parent interview, as well as in completing behavior rating forms. Often, if the concerns are serious enough, insurance companies will cover the cost of a psychological evaluation under your child's mental health benefits. Be careful to ask about your benefits, though, because some companies allow only a certain amount of coverage for the year for all mental health services, meaning that you may run out of benefits for things such as your child's psychotherapy. Remember, you can obtain an evaluation of your child's emotional and behavioral functioning through the public school system. The school will not likely refer to the testing as "psychological"; rather, it is usually called "emotional/behavioral testing." Often, though, an outside evaluation will be more thorough and can provide a diagnosis when appropriate.

As for how to talk to your child about this kind of evaluation, usually she will have a sense that something is not working right for her in her life, whether it's her mood, behavior, or something else. If you explain that the evaluation will help figure out why she is feeling so worried or angry or sad and suggest ways to help her feel better, she may actually be eager to go. It may also help when you tell her that the kinds of tests she'll be doing don't have right or wrong answers; she just needs to be honest about what she thinks and feels.

Sometimes older kids are worried about who will see the results of the testing; if you are paying for the evaluation with your insurance or out of pocket, you can reassure her that only you and her doctor(s) will see the report. If the school system does the testing or pays for an independent evaluation, however, you will not be able to give her this reassurance, as they will receive the results as well.

The Testing's Complete: Now What Do I Do?

Typically, if any of the disorders or problems discussed here are diagnosed by a medical or mental health professional, responsible follow-up care includes some form of treatment. (See the sidebar "Things to Keep in Mind after You Receive the Report" in Chapter Six.) For children with depression or anxiety, individual psychotherapy is often recommended. Kids who have ODD or CD will often be referred for individual therapy, and behavior management or parent guidance will be recommended for the parents. Children and teenagers with eating disorders may need to be stabilized medically first; then individual and family therapy is usually needed. Group therapy has also proven helpful to young people with eating disorders, self-injurious behaviors such as cutting, and even general depression and anxiety. The type and length of therapy will vary depending on factors such as the particular clinician, the child, the severity and type of problem, and, sadly, insurance coverage. Most insurance plans cover approximately eight to ten initial sessions, but it is then time-consuming for the therapist to obtain approval for more sessions and often costly to you, as coverage tends to be less the more sessions you use.

Though many childhood mental health concerns respond to therapy alone, some children will simply not improve or not improve enough without the addition of medication to the treatment plan. We have seen hundreds of children and adolescents whose lives changed

What Should I Tell My Child about the Diagnosis?

For the majority of school-age kids, we recommend talking to them about the diagnosis in age-appropriate terms. Many children often feel great relief in knowing that there is a reason or cause for their distress and that it actually has a name. By creating an open environment for discussing feelings and behavior, you will promote your child's well-being and recovery. If your child is already working with a therapist or if one has been recommended, it will be helpful for that clinician to discuss what it means to have depression or obsessive–compulsive disorder and what can be done to help. The therapist can also help your child figure out constructive ways to talk about his difficulties with peers and teachers if necessary (e.g., they want to know why he has missed a lot of school). One message that is really important for kids to get is that they are not alone in feeling the way they do and that it is common for people to sometimes get depressed, feel anxious, and so forth. Books that reinforce this idea are available for kids to read themselves, and many resources for parents are also available (see the end of the chapter). By taking care of yourself, you set a good example for your children and let them know that it's OK to get help.

for the better dramatically when they took medicine in conjunction with psychotherapy, and as a result, their families' lives improved as well. In certain cases, such as children with psychotic disorders, medication is the first intervention indicated. For most other concerns, though, some type of therapy will be recommended first, and the need for medication will be assessed by the therapist as treatment progresses. For helpful references on kids and psychiatric medication, see the Resources that follow.

Resources

Books for Parents

Alexander, D. (1999). *Children changed by trauma: A healing guide.* Oakland, CA: New Harbinger.

Berg, F. (2001). *Children and teens afraid to eat: Helping youth in today's weight-obsessed world.* Hettinger, ND: Healthy Weight Network.

Boskind-White, M., & White, W. (2000). *Bulimia/anorexia: The binge–purge cycle and self-starvation*. New York: Norton.

Claude-Pierre, P. (1997). *The secret language of eating disorders*. New York: Vintage.

Conterio, K., & Lader, W. (1998). *Bodily harm*. New York: Hyperion Press.

Dacey, J., & Fiore, L. (2000). *Your anxious child* San Francisco: Jossey-Bass.

Demitri, F., Papolos, M., & Papolos, J. (2002). *The bipolar child: The definitive and reassuring guide to childhood's most misunderstood disorder* (rev. and expanded ed.). New York: Broadway Books.

Greene, R. (2001). *The explosive child: A new approach for understanding and parenting easily frustrated, chronically inflexible children*. New York: HarperCollins.

Koplewicz, H. (2002). *More than moody: Recognizing and treating adolescent depression*. New York: Putnam.

Lynn, G. (2000). *Survival strategies for parenting children with bipolar disorder: Innovative parenting and counseling techniques for helping children with bipolar disorder and the conditions that may occur with it*. London: Jessica Kingsley.

Mondimone, F. (2002). *Adolescent depression: A guide for parents* Johns Hopkins University Press.

Rapee, R., Spence, S., Cobham, V., & Wignall, A. (2000). *Helping your anxious child: A step by step guide for parents* Oakland, CA: New Harbinger.

Riley, D. (2000). *The depressed child: A parent's guide to rescuing kids*. New York: Cooper Square Press.

Riley, D. (2002). *The defiant child: A parent's guide to oppositional defiant disorder*. Cutten, CA: Taylor.

Schaub, A. (2002). *New family interventions and associated research in psychosis* New York: Springer.

Wilens, T. (1999). *Straight talk about psychiatric medications for kids*. New York: Guilford Press.

Books for Children

Cracy, E., & Megale, M. (1996). *Mommy don't go* (Children's Problem Solving Book). Mahwah, NJ: Paulist Press.

McCoy, K., & Wibbelsman, C. (1996). *Life happens: A teenager's guide to friends, failure, sexuality, love, rejection, addiction, peer pressure, families, loss, depression, change and other challenges*. New York: Perigree Press.

Porter, D. (1999). *Taming monster moments*. Paulist Press.

Sederman, M., Epstein, S., & Brooks, K. S. (2003). *The magic box: When parents can't be there to tuck you in*. Washington, DC: Magination Press.

Organizations/Web Sites

American Anorexia Bulimia Association
165 West 46th Street, Suite 1108
New York, NY 10036
www.aabainc.org

Anxiety Disorders Association of America
11900 Parklawn Drive, Suite 100
Rockville, MD 20852
www.adaa.org

The Child and Adolescent Bipolar Foundation (CABF)
1187 Wilmette Avenue, PMB #331
Wilmette, IL 60091
www.cabf.org

Federation of Families for Children's Mental Health
1021 Prince Street
Alexandria, VA 22314
www.ffcmh.org

National Depressive and Manic–Depressive Association
730 North Franklin Street, Suite 501
Chicago, IL 60610
www.ndmda.org

National Foundation for Depression/Depressive Illness
P.O. Box 2257
New York, NY 10116
www.depression.org

The Obsessive Compulsive Foundation
P.O. Box 70
Milford, CT 06460
www.ocfoundation.org

Resources

Although we've listed resources at the end of Chapters 6 through 12, what follows are a variety of resources to provide additional information on various topics covered in this book.

Books

Adelizzi, J. U. (2001). *Parenting children with learning disabilities.* Westport, CT: Bergin & Garvey Press.

Anderson, W., Chitwood, S., & Hayden, D. (1997). *Negotiating the special education maze: A guide for parents and teachers* (3rd ed.). Bethesda, MD: Woodbine House.

Cicci, R. (1995). *What's wrong with me? Learning disabilities at home and at school.* Toronto, Canada: York Press.

Cutler, B. C. (1993). *You, your child, and "special" education: A guide for making the system work.* Baltimore: Brookes.

Faraone, S. V. (2003). *Straight talk about your child's mental health.* New York: Guilford Press.

Fisher, G., & Cummings, R. (1995). *When your child has LD (learning differences): A survival guide for parents.* Minneapolis, MN: Free Spirit Press.

Greene, R. (2001). *The explosive child: A new approach for understanding and parenting easily frustrated, chronically inflexible children.* New York: HarperCollins.

Hamacuchi, P. (2001). *Childhood speech, language and listening problems* (2nd ed.). New York: Wiley.

Healy, J. (1994). *Your child's growing mind: A guide to learning and brain development from birth to adolescence.* New York: Doubleday.

Kent, D., & Quinlan, K. (1996). *Extraordinary people with disabilities.* Minneapolis, MN: Children's Press.

Kopelwicz, H. W. (1996). *It's nobody's fault: New hope and help for difficult children and their parents.* New York: Times Books.

Kranowitz, C. (1998). *The out of sync child: Recognizing and coping with sensory integration dysfunction.* New York: Perigree.

Latham, P. S., & P. H. Latham. (1997). *Attention deficit disorder and the law* (2nd ed.). Washington, DC: JKL Communications.

Levine, M. (1990). *Keeping a head in school.* Cambridge, MA: Educators Publishing Service.

Levine, M. (1993). *All kinds of minds.* Cambridge, MA: Educators Publishing Service.

Levine, M. (2002). *Educational care* (2nd ed.). Cambridge, MA: Educators Publishing Service.

Levine, M. (2003). *A mind at a time.* New York: Simon & Schuster.

Levine, M., & Levine, M. (1992). *All kinds of minds: A young student's book about learning abilities and learning disabilities.* Cambridge, MA: Educators Publishing Service.

Lyon, G. R., & Krasnegor, N. A. (1996). *Attention, memory, and executive function.* Baltimore: Brookes.

Mastropicri, M., & T. Scruggs. (1999). *Teaching students ways to remember: Strategies for learning mnemonically.* Cambridge, MA: Brookline Books.

Rutter, M., & Rutter, M. (1993). *Developing minds.* New York: HarperCollins.

Sedita, J. (1989). *Landmark study skills guide.* Prides Crossing, MA: Landmark Foundation.

Siegel, L. M. (2001). *The complete IEP guide: How to advocate for your special ed child* (2nd ed.). Berkeley, CA: Nolo.

Shure, M. B. (1994). *Raising a thinking child.* New York: Pocket Books.

Turecki, S., & Tonner, L. (2000). *The difficult child* (2nd ed.). New York: Bantam Doubleday Dell.

Vail, P. (1987). *Smart kids with school problems.* New York: Dutton.

Weiss, G., & Hechtman, L. T. (1993). *Hyperactive children grown up* (2nd ed.). New York: Guilford Press.

Wilens, T. (2001). *Straight talk about psychiatric medications for kids.* New York: Guilford Press.

Wright, P., & Wright, P. (2001). *From emotions to advocacy: The special education survival guide.* Hartfield, VA: Harbour House Law Press.

Organizations

The American Academy of Child and Adolescent Psychiatry
3615 Wisconsin Avenue, NW
Washington, DC 20016-3007
Phone: 800-333-7636
www.aacap.org

American Association on Mental Retardation
444 North Capital Street, NW
Suite 846
Washington, DC 20001-1512
800-424-3688
www.aamr.org

The Child and Adolescent Bipolar Foundation (CABF)
1187 Wilmette Avenue PMB#331
Wilmette, IL 60091
847-256-8525
www.cabf.org

Council for Disability Rights
205 West Randolph, Suite 1645
Chicago, IL 60606
312-444-1967
www.disabilityrights.org

Council for Exceptional Children
1110 North Glebe Road
Suite 100
Arlington, VA 22201-5704
888-CEC-SPED
www.cec.sped.org

ERIC Clearinghouse on Disabilities and Gifted Education
1110 North Glebe Road
Arlington, VA 22201-5704
1800-328-0272
www.ericec.org

National Depressive and Manic–Depressive Association
730 North Franklin Street
Suite 501
Chicago, IL 60610-3526
800-826-3632; 312-642-0049
www.ndmda.org

National Foundation for Depressive Illness
PO Box 2257
New York, NY 10116
800-248-4344
www.depression.org

National Institute of Mental Health
Child Psychiatry Branch
5600 Fishers Lane
Rockville, MD 20857
301-443-4513

Web Sites

About Our Kids
www.aboutourkids.org
   —A child and adolescent mental health and parenting resource

Advocacy Institute
www.advocacyinstitute.org

All Kinds of Minds
www.allkindsofminds.org

Child Advocate
www.childadvocate.net

Child and Family Webpage
www.cfw.tufts.edu/index.html

Children with Disabilities
www.childrenwithdisabilities.ncjrs.org

Council for Children with Behavioral Disorders
www.ccbd.net

Keep Kids Learning
www.keepkidslearning.org

Kid Source on Line
www.kidsource.com

Learning Disabilities Association of America
www.ldanatl.org

Mental Health Infosource
www.mhsource.com

Misunderstood Minds
www.pbs.org/wgbh/misunderstoodminds

National Center for Learning Disabilities
www.ld.org

National Mental Health Association
www.nmha.org

Parents and Teachers of Explosive Kids
www.explosivekids.org

Index

About the Authors

Ellen Braaten, PhD, is the track director of the Child/Adult and Neuropsychology training programs at Massachusetts General Hospital and is on the faculty of Harvard Medical School. Dr. Braaten is a staff psychologist at the Massachusetts General Hospital's Psychology Assessment Center, where she specializes in child neuropsychology. She has authored numerous scientific papers and chapters on children with ADHD, depression, anxiety, and learning disabilities. She resides with her husband and two children, Hannah and Peter, in the Boston area.

Gretchen Felopulos, PhD, is a licensed clinical psychologist on the Massachusetts General Hospital staff in Child Psychiatry and in its Psychology Assessment Center. She is also on the faculty of Harvard Medical School and has a private practice in Lexington, Massachusetts. In addition to her specialization in pediatric neuropsychology and psychological testing, Dr. Felopulos provides psychotherapy to children as well as parental guidance. She is a primary supervisor for psychology interns studying the process of testing, and she teaches many seminars each year to interns and residents on the topic of children and testing. She, her husband, and their three children live in suburban Boston.